Domestic and Sexual Violenc and Abuse

Domestic violence, childhood sexual abuse, rape and sexual assault, and sexual exploitation through prostitution, pornography and trafficking can have many significant adverse impacts on a survivor's health and wellbeing, in the short, medium and long term.

Taking a life-course approach, the book explores what is known about appropriate treatment responses to those who have experienced, and those who perpetrate, domestic and sexual violence and abuse. The book also examines key factors that are important in understanding how and why different groups experience heightened risks of domestic and sexual violence and abuse, namely: gender and sexuality; race and culture; disability; and abuse by professionals.

Drawing together results from specially commissioned research, the views of experts by experience, experts by profession and the published research literature, the book argues that sufficient is already known to delineate an appropriate public health framework, encompassing primary, secondary and tertiary prevention, to successfully tackle the important public health issue represented by domestic and sexual violence and abuse. *Domestic and Sexual Violence and Abuse* equips health and social care professionals and services with the skills and knowledge to identify and respond to the needs of affected individuals with a view to prevention and early intervention.

Catherine Itzin was Emerita Professor in Mental Health Policy, University of Lincoln, UK until her death on 9 March 2010.

Ann Taket is Professor of Health and Social Exclusion in the School of Health and Social Development, Deakin University, Australia.

Sarah Barter-Godfrey is Lecturer in the School of Health and Social Development, Deakin University, Australia.

Domestic and Sexual Violence and Abuse

Tackling the health and mental health effects

Catherine Itzin, Ann Taket and Sarah Barter-Godfrey

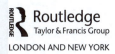
Routledge
Taylor & Francis Group

LONDON AND NEW YORK

First published 2010
by Routledge
2 Park Square, Milton Park, Abingdon, Oxon, OX14 4RN

Simultaneously published in the USA and Canada
by Routledge
270 Madison Avenue, New York, NY 10016

Routledge is an imprint of the Taylor & Francis Group, an informa
business

Typeset in Sabon by RefineCatch Limited, Bungay, Suffolk.

Printed and bound in Great Britain by TJ International Ltd,
Padstow, Cornwall

British Library Cataloguing in Publication Data
A catalogue record for this book is available from the British Library

Library of Congress Cataloging in Publication Data
   Domestic and sexual violence and abuse : tackling the health and
     mental health effects / edited by Catherine Itzin, Ann Taket, and
     Sarah Barter-Godfrey.
       p. ; cm.
   1. Family violence. 2. Adult child abuse victims—Mental health. 3.
   Abused children—Mental health. 4. Sexual abuse victims—Mental
   health. I. Itzin, Catherine, 1944– II. Taket, A. R. (Ann R.) III.
   Barter-Godfrey, Sarah.
   [DNLM: 1. Adult Survivors of Child Abuse—psychology. 2.
   Domestic Violence—psychology. 3. Mental Health. 4. Sex
   Offenses—psychology. WM 167 D668 2011]
   RC569.5.F3D648 2011
   362.82 2—dc22
   2010012835

ISBN13: 978–0–415–55531–9 (hbk)
ISBN13: 978–0–415–55532–6 (pbk)
ISBN13: 978–0–203–84220–1 (ebk)

Contents

Acknowledgements

First of all, we would like to acknowledge and salute the courage, inventiveness and creativity of all those who have been victims and survivors of domestic and sexual violence and abuse. Their considerable achievements are woven throughout the fabric of this book, and the work that has led to the writing of this book would not have been possible without their generosity in sharing their experiences.

The work of the VVAPP programme, and the production of this book, would also not have been possible without the very active involvement of the different expert groups involved in advising the programme, both experts by profession and experts by experience, as well as those who participated in the different research components within the programme. Our thanks go out to all of them.

Disclaimer

This book discusses the results of research commissioned by the Department of Health and the Home Office under the Victims of Violence and Abuse Prevention Programme (VVAPP). The views expressed are those of the authors and are not necessarily shared by the Department of Health.

Dedication

Catherine Itzin-Borowy

1944–2010

All of us involved in the writing of this book would like to dedicate it to the memory of Catherine Itzin-Borowy.

The book was originally Catherine's initiative, and we were fortunate enough to have her contribution throughout the major period of its writing. Sadly she died in the last stages of the finalisation of the manuscript.

Catherine was a tireless advocate for better services to meet the needs of those whose lives have been affected by domestic and sexual violence and abuse. Within the Victims of Violence and Abuse Prevention Programme which she directed, and which formed the impetus for this book, she worked to ensure that the voices of those who have experienced violence and abuse helped to shape the scope and direction of the programme, and were present at all stages within the programme's work.

Catherine's passion and commitment for the work she was involved in was evident to all who knew her. She leaves behind her a substantial and important body of feminist work on sexual abuse, pornography and domestic abuse in her books and papers. Many of us have enjoyed the privilege of working with her at different points throughout her life. She will be very sadly missed by us and by all in the sexual and domestic violence fields.

List of authors

Jackie Barron works in the National Office of Women's Aid, the UK national domestic violence charity working with women and children.

Sarah Barter-Godfrey is a Lecturer in the School of Health and Social Development, Deakin University, Australia.

Richard Curen is Chief Executive of Respond, UK, the organisation supporting people with learning disabilities, their families, carers and professionals affected by trauma and abuse.

Jalna Hanmer is a Professor in the School of Health and Social Sciences, University of Sunderland, UK.

Nicola Harwin, CBE, is Chief Executive of Women's Aid, the UK national domestic violence charity working with women and children.

Marianne Hester is Professor of Gender, Violence and International Policy in the School for Policy Studies, University of Bristol, UK.

Catherine Itzin was Emerita Professor in Mental Health Policy, University of Lincoln, UK until her death on 9 March 2010.

Ruth Marchant is a co-Director of Triangle, an independent organisation in the UK that works directly with children and families, gives expert opinion to the courts and teaches and advises parents and professionals.

Meena Patel works for Southall Black Sisters, London, UK, a not-for-profit organisation, that provides a comprehensive service to black (Asian and African-Caribbean) women experiencing violence and abuse.

Hannana Siddiqui is the Coordinator and Policy Worker, Southall Black Sisters, London, UK, a not-for-profit organisation, that provides a comprehensive service to black (Asian and African-Caribbean) women experiencing violence and abuse.

Valerie Sinason is the Director of the Clinic for Dissociative Studies, and consultant research psychotherapist at St George's Hospital, London, UK.

Ann Taket is Professor of Health and Social Exclusion in the School of Health and Social Development, Deakin University, Australia.

List of illustrations

Figures

Tables

Case studies

List of acronyms

ACPO	Association of Chief Police Officers
ADHD	Attention Deficit Hyperactivity Disorder
BACP	British Association for Counselling and Psychotherapy
BCS	British Crime Survey
BME	Black and Minority Ethnic
BSL	British Sign Language
CAFCASS	Children and Family Court Advisory and Support Service
CAMHS	Child and Adolescent Mental Health Services (UK)
CBT	Cognitive behavioural therapy
CDRP	Crime and Disorder Reduction Partnership
CPS	Crown Prosecution Service
CROP	Coalition for the Removal of Pimping
CSA	Child sexual abuse
CTS	Conflict Tactics Scale
DCSF	Department for Children, Schools and Families
DES	Department for Education and Skills
DH	Department of Health
DRC	Disability Rights Commission
DV	domestic violence and abuse
EDCM	Every Disabled Child Matters
EMDR	Eye Movement Desensitisation and Reprocessing
EPM	Extreme pornographic material
FCO	Foreign and Commonwealth Office
HO	Home Office
HPA	hypothalamic–pituitary–adrenal
IBS	irritable bowel syndrome
IPA	Intimate partner abuse
IPD	Institute for the Psychotherapy of Disability
IPV	Intimate partner violence
LAA	Local Area Agreement
LGBT	Lesbian, gay, bisexual and transgender
LHRH	Luteinizing Hormone Releasing Hormone
MST	Multisystemic Therapy

N6   a qualitative data analysis package
NCCWCH National Collaborating Centre for Women's and Children's
              Health
NCIPC   National Center for Injury Prevention and Control (US)
NGO   Non-governmental organisation
NHS   National Health Service
NICE   National Institute for Clinical Excellence
NIMHE   National Institute for Mental Health in England
NSPCC   National Society of Prevention of Cruelty to Children (UK)
OCD   Obsessive compulsive disorder
OPCS   Office of Population Censuses and Surveys (UK)
PHSE   Personal, Health and Social Education
POPAN   Prevention of Professional Abuse Network (UK)
PTSD   Post-traumatic stress disorder
SARC   Sexual Assessment Referral Centre
SBS   Southall Black Sisters
SOTP   Sex Offender Treatment Programmes
SPSS   Statistical Package for the Social Sciences
SSE   sign-supported English
SSRI   selective serotonin reuptake inhibitor
UKP   United Kingdom Parliament
UN   United Nations
US NVAW United States National Violence Against Women survey
USCCB   United States Conference of Catholic Bishops
VIMH   Violence Induced Mental Handicap
VVAPP   Victims of Violence and Abuse Prevention Programme
WHO   World Health Organization
WWDA   Women with Disabilities Australia

Part I

Setting the scene

Collaboration is at the heart of this work – across government, across all sectors, all professionals and disciplines – essentially informed by the strong voice of victims and survivors, of all ages and from all backgrounds. The VVAPP is the central vehicle for the development of policy and consensus on the needs and interventions required by victims, survivors and abusers. The ultimate challenge will be the transformation of practice on the ground.

Society as a whole needs to acknowledge and accept the endemic nature of violence and abuse but, in particular, we – as politicians, policy makers and professionals – need to assume our collective responsibility to address it, reduce its prevalence and ultimately work towards its eradication.

(Then Minister of State for Public Health Caroline Flint, in the press release for the launch of the Victims of Violence and Abuse Prevention Programme, 26 November 2006 (at http://www.dh.gov.uk/en/Publicationsandstatistics/ Pressreleases/DH_4136528 accessed 29 November 2009))

1 Introduction
The Victims of Violence and Abuse Prevention Programme (VVAPP) and its work

This single chapter provides a summary of the VVAPP programme, the relevant policy backgrounds (in particular health and criminal justice) and research content of the programme. It explores the achievements of the UK Government in addressing the needs of victims/survivors of domestic and sexual violence and abuse.

Domestic and sexual violence and abuse: a major public health issue

Domestic and sexual violence and abuse affects a very substantial minority of the population. It is largely women, and children of both sexes, who are affected, but men are also raped and experience domestic violence. Child physical, emotional or sexual abuse and neglect and domestic violence are causal factors in the mental and physical ill-health of children, adolescents and adults and affect a significant proportion throughout their lives. The high costs in prevalence and economic burden on health and social care services and the criminal justice system have pushed these issues up the policy agenda. They have figured prominently in Department of Health (DH) policy on mental health, child health, women's health, and public health, and in wider government policy on child poverty, victims and witnesses, social exclusion, human trafficking and safeguarding children (see Appendix 1). During the life of VVAPP from 2004 to 2008 they were also the focus of cross-government working with the Department of Health, Department for Children, Schools and Families and the Home Office through the (then) Inter-ministerial Groups on Domestic Violence and Sexual Offending in the wider context of new legislation on domestic violence, sexual offences and mental health.

Intimate Partner Abuse (IPA) is a major public health problem and one of the most widespread human rights violations. It remains under-acknowledged in all European countries, as it is throughout the world. Worldwide, 10–50 per cent of women report having been hit or physically assaulted by an intimate partner at some time in their lives (Heise et al. 1999). In a large international study (24,097 interviews in total) across 15 sites in 10 countries

Garcia-Moreno and colleagues (2006) find reported lifetime prevalence of physical or sexual partner violence, or both, varied from 15 per cent to 71 per cent, with two sites having a prevalence of less than 25 per cent, seven between 25 per cent and 50 per cent, and six between 50 per cent and 75 per cent. Between 4 per cent and 54 per cent of respondents reported physical or sexual partner violence, or both, in the past year. Intimate partner violence occurs in all countries, and throughout society in each country, irrespective of social, economic, religious or cultural group (Garcia-Moreno et al. 2006; Heise et al. 1999; Krug et al. 2002; WHO 1997).

In the UK, 23 per cent (1 in 4) of women aged 16–59 has been physically assaulted by a current or former partner. Two women are killed every week in the UK by a current or former partner (Mirlees-Black 1999). Similar results are shown in studies elsewhere in Europe on the prevalence of violence against women (Heiskanen and Piispa 2001, Jaspard et al. 2003, Lundgren et al. 2002, Müller and Schröttle 2004). The health effects on those directly experiencing domestic violence include:

- Physical health: injuries from the assault, chronic physical health problems, e.g. IBS, backache and headaches (Campbell 2002);
- Reproductive health: increased unintended pregnancies, terminations (Gazmararian et al. 2000), low birth weight babies (Murphy et al. 2001), and pregnancy-associated deaths (Shadigian and Bauer 2005);
- Sexual health: higher rates of sexually transmitted infections, including HIV (Garcia-Moreno and Watts 2000);
- Mental health: higher rates of depression, anxiety, Post-Traumatic Stress Disorder, self-harm and suicide (Campbell 2002; Golding 1999; Romito et al. 2005; Silva et al. 1997).

Children growing up with domestic abuse are 30–60 per cent more likely to experience child abuse themselves (Edleson 1999b; Hester et al. 2007; Humphreys and Thiara 2002). A Department of Health study of 44 children on the child protection register found domestic violence in two-fifths of the child sexual abuse cases and in three-fifths of the cases of physical abuse, neglect and emotional abuse (Farmer and Owen 1995). Children who witness abuse exhibit symptoms of sleep disturbance, poor school performance, emotional detachment, stammering, suicide attempts, aggressive, and disruptive behaviour (Knapp 1998; McWilliams and McKiernan 1993; Shankleman et al. 2001; Stark and Flitcraft 1988). Children who witness domestic abuse learn to accept abuse as an appropriate method of conflict resolution and are more likely to repeat patterns in adulthood (Rosenberg and Rossman 1990). The presence of IPA against women is a risk factor for abuse and ill-health among children and youth (Hedin 2000). Children who experience abuse and neglect are at significant risk for problems in later life across several socioeconomic domains, including income, employment status, and, healthcare coverage (Zielinski 2009).

The costs of IPA in the US exceed $5.8 billion each year (NCIPC 2003). The cost to the NHS in the UK for physical injuries alone resulting from IPA is approx £1.2 billion a year (Walby 2004). Similarly high figures are provided by studies in other European countries such as Switzerland (Godenzi and Yodanis 1998), the Netherlands (Korf et al. 1997) and Finland (Heiskanen and Piispa 2001).

Attitudes to abuse in general and IPA in particular are known to vary across different linguistic, cultural and religious communities and according to different contextual variables including education (Glick et al. 2002; Hagemann-White 2001; Haj-Yahia 2002; Herzog 2004; Krahe et al. 2005; Nayak et al. 2003, Pan et al. 2003; Simon et al. 2001; Vanya 2001).

IPA is experienced within all types of relationships, both same-sex and heterosexual (Krug et al. 2002) Although approximately one in seven men in the UK report experiencing physical assault by a current or former partner (Mirlees-Black 1999), these incidents are generally less serious than those reported by women, and men are less likely to be injured, frightened or seek medical care (DH 2005b; Dobash and Dobash 2003, 2004). Although domestic violence can take place in any intimate relationship, including gay and lesbian partnerships, and abuse of men by female partners does occur, the great majority of IPA, and the most severe and chronic incidents, are perpetrated by men against women. The context and severity of violence by men against women makes domestic violence against women a much larger problem in public health terms (Krug et al. 2002; Taft et al. 2001; WHO 1997).

Community studies in the US and the UK have consistently identified 20–30 per cent of women and 5–10 per cent of men reporting sexual abuse in childhood. In the US, Finkelhor (1994) found in a meta-analysis of 19 prevalence studies 20 per cent of women and 10 per cent of men reporting child sexual abuse (CSA). In the UK, Kelly and colleagues (1991) found 21 per cent of women and 7 per cent of men reporting sexual abuse as a child, and the NSPCC study by Cawson et al. (2000) found 21 per cent of women and 11 per cent of men doing so. The NSPCC study also found high levels of physical and emotional abuse and neglect: frequent and severe emotional abuse experienced by 6 per cent of children; neglect defined as serious absence of care involving 6 per cent of children; 21 per cent of children subjected to physical violence regularly and 7 per cent experiencing severe physical abuse (Cawson et al. 2000). Co-occurrence is common, meaning multiple and more severe abuse for many individual children.

The British Crime Survey (2004–2005) found that 23 per cent of women and 3 per cent of men are subject to sexual victimisation in some form during their lifetime and 7 per cent of women and 0.5 per cent of men experienced rape or severe sexual assault in the previous year; 54 per cent of rapes were committed by a woman's partner (45 per cent) or ex-partner (9 per cent); in addition a further 35 per cent of rapists were known to their victim (e.g. date rape); only 11 per cent were stranger rapes (Finney 2006).

Repeat victimisation is common across all forms of domestic and sexual violence and abuse. Domestic violence typically escalates in frequency and severity over time (Krug et al. 2002), with the highest rate of revictimisation of any crime (Dodd et al. 2004; Stanko 2003). Most children who are sexually abused are repeatedly victimised whether the abuse is intra- or extra-familial. 'Predatory paedophiles' are known to abuse very substantial numbers of children during a 'lifetime's career' (Wyre 2000). Most adult rapists are also serial abusers whether it is intimate partner, date rape or stranger rape (Stanko 2003).

There are no prevalence data for domestic violence (DV) perpetrators, or rapists, or adult sex offenders against children, or for young people who sexually abuse. However, it is known that 20–30 per cent of sex offenders who are cautioned or convicted are under the age of 18 (Lovell 2002). Half of adult sex offenders report an 'adolescent onset of sexual deviance' (Abel et al. 1985).

There are significant criminal justice system costs associated with the crimes of domestic and sexual violence and abuse which, together with the costs of mental and physical ill health and its treatment, need to be taken into account from a public health perspective (Walby 2004). The health effects on victims of sexual violence and abuse include:

- Psychological and behavioural effects: PTSD, depression, suicide, sexual promiscuity, victim–perpetrator cycle, poor academic performance (Evans et al. 2005; Paolucci et al. 2001; Veltman and Browne 2001); and eating disorders (Smolak and Murnen 2002);
- Revictimisation (Classen et al. 2005) and intergenerational transmission (Bornstein 2005);
- HIV risk behaviour: unprotected sex, sex with multiple partners, sex trading and adult sexual revictimisation (Arriola et al. 2005);
- Reproductive health: adolescent pregnancy (Blinn-Pike et al. 2002); pregnancy, delivery, and early post partum difficulties (Leeners et al. 2006);
- Physical health: chronic pelvic pain (Latthe et al 2006); irritable bowel syndrome (Payne 2004).

In understanding domestic and sexual violence and abuse, Heise's 'ecological framework' for studying violence against women (Heise 1998) is used. This framework views violence and abuse as resulting from the complex interaction of a variety of factors, each of which operates on a variety of different levels. The framework distinguishes four different levels: individual, relationship, community and society. The individual level is defined as personality factors and events that occur within a person's lifetime that help to shape an individual's responses to situations and stresses. The second level, which is of the relationship, represents the immediate context in which violence and abuse takes place. The third level, community, includes the institutions and social structures, both formal and informal, in which relationships are embedded: neighbourhood, workplace, social networks and peer groups. The fourth level, society, or the 'macrosystem', is the economic and social environment, including cultural norms, defined as the set of commonly accepted cultural values, beliefs, and practices that permeate and govern a society.

Research has shown that exposure to domestic and sexual violence and abuse in the home is associated with being a victim or perpetrator of violence in adolescence and adulthood (Maxfield and Widom 1996). Normative beliefs about blame and responsibility for action for IPA do not always align; for example an American study found that although blame was placed mostly on assailants, victims were held either mutually or primarily responsible for taking action in 83 per cent of the cases (Taylor and Sorenson 2003). In addition, beliefs were influenced by victim and assailant gender and sexual orientation, as well as by situational factors. Burris and Jackson (1999) demonstrated, in the US context, that whether religion discourages or encourages attitudes to IPA may depend on who is being abused.

Definitions and cautions

This book refers to both violence and abuse consistently with reference to both domestic violence and sexual violence. This reflects actual differences in the nature of what is perpetrated. For example domestic violence includes physical and sexual violence in different forms, but also psychological and verbal abuse, and financial and economic control (being deprived of money and prevented from working) which would not correctly be conceptualised as violence.

Child sexual abuse not sexual violence is the terminology generally employed for the penetration of a child's genitals or anus or mouth by a penis or object. In fact, the Sexual Offences Act (UKP 2003) defines this as rape, so much of what is known as child sexual abuse is defined by law as rape and sexual assault. The sexual abuse, assault and rape of children which is photographed or videoed is increasingly referred to as child sexual abuse images rather than child pornography to emphasise that it involves the actual sexual abuse/assault/rape of a child. Similarly what was previously called child pornography on the computer or internet is now called online child sexual abuse images, some of which have been photographed and reproduced and some of which take place in 'real time'.

Within the book the terms 'victims' and 'survivors' are both used. This is to reflect the fact that violence and abuse involves victimisation perpetrated by a person who is usually physically and socially more powerful than the person they victimise, whether this is an adult abusing a child or another adult. Being victimised is always disempowering and there is a view that the use of the word 'victim' is also disempowering. However, using the term victim simply acknowledges that the person was victimised, and helps to make violence and abuse more visible in a societal context where this has not always been the case. The term survivor has been used out of respect for the many people who think of themselves as survivors, including the 130 member organisations of the Survivors Trust. It also reflects the enormity of victimisation: that such a child had to go into 'inner world survivor mode' to protect its very being, sanity and security. However, since most go on to do so much more than survive, the use of the word does not seem to do full justice to their achievements.

The term 'sex offenders' is used to refer to those who have committed sexual offences and been caught. Most sexual abusers never come into contact with the criminal justice system because they are not identified. The majority of child sexual abuse is not reported, hence the use of 'sexual abusers' to denote those individuals and to highlight them as potential recipients of preventive interventions in the health service or voluntary sector if they were identified and sufficient help were available. Historically and currently those who commit domestic violence have been referred to as 'perpetrators'. Most of them never come into contact with the criminal justice system either, because most women do not report domestic violence, but the word does not denote their criminal status.

For the purposes of this book intimate partner abuse (IPA) is defined as 'the physical, sexual, emotional and/or financial abuse of people who are, or have been, intimate partners – whether or not they are married or co-habiting – in order to maintain power and control over that person'. Abuse may continue after the partners have separated. A very important feature of this definition is the inclusion of the phrase 'in order to maintain power and control over that person'; this feature of coercive control distinguishes what is referred to as IPA (or intimate terrorism by some) from what has been labelled elsewhere as situational couple violence. Johnson (2008) provides a helpful analysis of the differences between these two distinctly different entities and explores the problems methodological and otherwise that have resulted from a failure to distinguish them.

Within the UK the term 'domestic violence' or 'domestic abuse' is often used instead of IPA; however, elsewhere in the English-speaking world (Australia and New Zealand in particular) the terms 'domestic violence' or 'domestic abuse' are used to refer to all violence/abuse in the family setting (including child abuse and elder abuse), i.e. not just to abuse involving an intimate partner, so the term IPA is used to remove the danger of confusion. This definition draws on a number of different sources, including the Beijing Platform for Action (UN 1995), the UN Declaration on the Elimination of Violence Against Women (UN 1996), the British Council (1999), and the World Report on Violence and Health (Krug et al. 2002).

Learning-disabled people

In some cases there are clear geographical differences in terminology; for example, the UK uses learning disability/learning disabled, Australia uses intellectual disability/intellectually disabled, and North America uses developmental disability/developmentally disabled. Throughout the book the UK usage is adopted and learning disability/learning disabled are the terms used.

The legislative and policy contexts

The legislative and policy landscape which frames responses to domestic and sexual violence and abuse is complex. Adequate responses to violence and abuse including prevention and early intervention involve a wide range of sectors in society: health; criminal justice; social care; education; employment; and housing to name but a few. A major challenge is in achieving the necessary high level of integration and coordination at all stages in the policy process, from development through to implementation, evaluation and re-development, and at and between all levels in society, from national, through regional to local levels of government and service provision. Relevant service-providing agencies span a similarly wide range of sectors, and include the statutory sector, the private sector and the third sector. The third sector is particularly significant as it is within this sector that much of the specialised services responding to the needs of victims and survivors have been shaped over decades.

Central to providing services in this area in the UK is the specialist voluntary sector comprising over 600 domestic violence services provided by Women's Aid, Refuge and other organisations, the 130 Survivors Trust services for adult victims and survivors of rape and sexual assault and sexual abuse in childhood, the 37 Rape Crisis Centres, and the hundreds of services provided by the major Children's Charities (NSPCC, Barnardo's and the Children's Society).

In this chapter some key aspects of the legislation and policy contexts within the UK are introduced. Although a comprehensive review is beyond the scope of this book, key pieces of legislation and policies are discussed in the later chapters.

Relevant legislation includes: the Sexual Offences Act (UKP 2003), the Domestic Violence Crime and Victims Act (UKP 2004), the Adoption and Children Act (UKP 2002) making domestic violence a significant harm for children, the Equality Act (UKP 2006), and a new offence of possession of extreme pornographic material in the Criminal Justice and Immigration Act (UKP 2008). Implementation of the legislation has been supported by Public Service Agreement targets and the publication of a wide range of policies and action plans on domestic violence, sexual violence and abuse, forced marriage, human trafficking, prostitution and a great deal more. Altogether there are over thirty key government policy initiatives to guide and support improvements in services for victims and more effective measures to stop abusers abusing (see Appendix 1).

In particular, it has become increasingly a priority to identify perpetrators and hold them accountable through a combination of prosecution and preventive interventions such as those set out in the Review of the Protection of Children from Sex Offenders report (HO 2007a) and Whittle, Bailey and Kurz (2006). The government has also produced a wide variety of delivery and action plans, including: the Violent Crime Action Plan (HO 2008); the first Domestic Violence Delivery Plan (HO 2005a), and its successors, up to the plan for 2009/2010 (HO 2009a); the National Sexual Violence and Abuse Action Plan (HM Government 2007), the UK Action Plan on Human Trafficking (HO 2007b); and set up a Taskforce on the Health Aspects of Violence against Women and Girls in May 2009. All of these were developed by government officials working closely with key stakeholders from statutory, voluntary and criminal justice sectors, overseen at that time by Inter-Departmental Ministerial Groups on Domestic Violence, Sexual Offending and Human Trafficking.

Significant publications to support continuing implementation of policies in the area include:

- National Institute for Clinical Excellence Guideline on Self Harm (NICE 2004); Responding to Domestic Abuse: A Handbook for Health Professionals (DH 2005b), which includes discussion of routine clinical enquiry about domestic abuse in antenatal care, accident and emergency departments, and other healthcare settings;
- Improving Safety, Reducing Harm, Children, Young People and Domestic Violence: A practical toolkit for front-line practitioners, produced by the Greater London Domestic Violence Project (Sharpen 2009);
- National Institute for Clinical Excellence's guidelines on when to suspect child maltreatment (NCCWCH 2009);
- National Institute for Clinical Excellence's public health guidance on promoting children's social and emotional well-being in primary education (NICE, 2008);
- National Institute for Clinical Excellence's public health guidance on promoting children's social and emotional well-being in secondary education (NICE 2009);
- Violence Against Women and Girls Strategy (HO 2009b).

These are discussed in more detail in the chapters that follow.

The VVAPP programme

The Department of Health and National Institute for Mental Health 'Victims of Violence and Abuse Prevention Programme' (VVAPP) was established under the direction of Professor Catherine Itzin in partnership with the Home Office and launched by Department of Health and Home Office Ministers at a National Domestic Violence Conference in October 2004 and a National Sexual Violence Conference in October 2005. The programme was in partnership with the Home Office's then Children and

Youth Justice Team, Victims Unit, Sexual Crime Reduction Team, Criminal Law Policy Unit and Domestic Violence Unit, and with the Department for Children, Schools and Families Safeguarding team. The VVAPP programme guide *Tackling the Health and Mental Health Effects of Domestic and Sexual Violence and Abuse* (Itzin 2006) was launched by the DH Public Health Minister in 2006.

This book draws on the research projects conducted within the VVAPP (discussed later in this chapter) in the context of government legislation and policy development. It covers domestic violence, childhood sexual abuse, rape and sexual assault, and sexual exploitation through prostitution, pornography and trafficking as it affects victims, survivors and abusers, including children, adolescents and adults, both male and female. The book reports findings from this research which covers:

- What is known about the sexual and domestic violence and abuse experienced by those affected (nature, extent, effects, needs);
- What is known to work in their treatment and care;
- What is required to protect victims from abuse with a focus on safety and risk management;
- What can be done to stop abusers abusing.

The aim of the VVAPP, its research and its publications was to equip professionals and services to identify and respond to the needs of affected individuals with a view to the prevention of the abuse occurring, to prevention and reduction (through early intervention) of its adverse effects, and appropriate therapeutic responses to adverse effects.

The VVAPP was advised by 150 leading experts in six expert groups and a panel of specialist advisers comprising leading academics and professionals from all relevant disciplines (including psychiatry, psychology, psychoanalysis and social work) and sectors, including domestic and sexual violence voluntary sector services, NHS, local authority children's services, criminal justice system service providers and Royal Colleges and professional bodies. The six expert groups were for: adult domestic violence victims, survivors and perpetrators; child victims of domestic violence and child sexual abuse; adolescent and adult sexual abusers and offenders; adult victims of rape and sexual assault; adult survivors of childhood sexual abuse; and adult, adolescent and child victims of prostitution, pornography and trafficking.

The VVAPP was divided into ten separate programme areas, necessary in order to adequately explore the complexity of violence and abuse within the programme, see Figure 1.1. Part II of this book offers a different view into the programme areas, by discussing in three separate chapters (3, 4 and 5 respectively), different stages in the life-course: childhood, adolescence and adulthood.

- Sexually abused children
- Child victims of domestic violence
- All victims/survivors of sexual exploitation in prostitution, pornography and trafficking (child, adolescent and adult)
- Children and young people who display sexually inappropriate behaviour or who sexually abuse other young people, children or adults
- Young people who perpetrate domestic violence
- Adult victims/survivors of rape and sexual assault
- Adult survivors of childhood sexual abuse
- Adult victims/survivors of domestic violence
- Adult perpetrators of domestic violence
- Adult sexual offenders

Figure 1.1 The ten programme areas in the VVAPP.

The VVAPP research programme

A number of separate research projects were commissioned to complement each other and to provide a triangulation of findings and evidence. One of these was a systematic review of reviews of the research literature published between January 2000 and April 2007 across all groups in the programme that examined epidemiology, impact, therapeutic interventions, protection and prevention. The literature identified in the review is used within this book, supplemented by the considerable volume of literature published since April 2007.

The programme also commissioned a Delphi expert consultation (Taket and Barter-Godfrey 2006) involving 285 individuals/organisations including leading academics and professionals from all disciplines, service providers from all sectors and organisations representing mental health services users. The Delphi thus included experts by both profession and experience. The Delphi consultation covered principles, values and core beliefs; theoretical models and therapeutic approaches; treatments; prevention; managing safety and risk; training; overcoming obstacles and improving outcomes. Its methods are described further below, and its findings are drawn out throughout Part II of this book.

The Violence and Abuse Care Pathways Mapping Project was developed in collaboration with victims and survivors of extreme and chronic abuse, and organisations providing preventive interventions with abusers. These included learning-disabled people and physically disabled people, and the experience of those from black and minority ethnic communities. Its methods are described further below and its findings are drawn on in Parts II and III of this book.

The Delphi consultation

This Delphi consultation was undertaken to identify where there is and is not consensus among experts about what is known and what works in the treatment and care of people affected by child sexual abuse, domestic violence and abuse, and rape and sexual assault. While helping to identify areas of agreement and disagreement about effective mental health service responses, the consultation aimed to support the evidence base derived from the literature review. The consultation covered the ten different areas within the programme (defined by different types of victim/survivor and abuser/perpetrator), see Figure 1.1.

Round 1 of the consultation posed a set of mainly open questions for each of the above 10 programme areas in turn. The questions covered seven broad topics: principles and core beliefs; effective interventions; managing safety and risk; training; prevention; improving outcomes; addressing obstacles. The actual questions are contained in Appendix 2. Participants in the consultation were asked to answer on the basis of their experience. Responses were accepted from individuals or organisations. No anonymous responses were allowed (the ethics clearance involved seeking explicit consent to participation, and successive rounds of the Delphi consultation required mailing out to the same group that responded in the first round). Respondents were invited to provide responses in relation to each of the programme areas in which they considered they had expertise.

Responses to Round 1 were anonymised before entry into N6 (a qualitative data analysis package) for analysis of qualitative comments. Analysis of qualitative responses received was carried out using multiple coders, repeated rounds of coding and code development, and a variety of consistency cross-checks in order to identify the range of different positions present in the responses, and to group and structure them. Within the report of Round 1 a detailed analysis of responses was provided in relation to therapeutic and treatment interventions. This category includes all interventions aimed at healing or ameliorating the effects of violence or abuse on victims/survivors, or at directly modifying violent or abusive behaviour. A high-level synthesis was provided in relation to the other areas covered in the Delphi. The emphasis in the Round 1 report was on reporting back the range of positions found in the responses and identifying areas of consensus and areas where there was a lack of consensus. The different positions were fed back in the form of statements (derived directly from Round 1 responses) on which rating and comment were invited in Round 2.

In analysing Round 2, SPSS (Statistical Package for the Social Sciences) was utilised to analyse responses to the statements. The comments were analysed separately in order to identify any additional positions, these were then fed back in the report of Round 2. Comments in relation to the different therapeutic approaches were included verbatim in most instances. Comments were numbered so that all respondents could refer to them if they wished in expressing their response in the final round, Round 3. In Round 3, respondents were invited to assess/reassess the different statements and positions, having seen the overall distribution of responses and read the comments of the other respondents from Round 2. Further comments were also invited.

The consultation was carried out to a very tight timetable, within a strictly limited budget. This adversely affected response rates, although the rates reported below are very good in the circumstances and adequate for the analysis presented here. Limitations of time and resource also constrained the analysis that it was possible to carry out. In addition, in relation to some of the 10 programme areas, the number of respondents on particular points or statements was small (under five) and in some cases only two or three. The timescale for the consultation meant that it was not possible to consider more than three rounds. Given the complexity of the issues addressed (and the breadth of the consultation), it is perhaps not surprising that many areas remained where consensus was not reached; at least part of this may have been due to the limitation to three rounds.

Participation was invited from all the different constituencies involved in the VVAPP programme, experts by both experience and profession. Participants were recruited through a variety of sources: VVAPP specialist advisers; members of the VVAPP expert groups and their nominees; Royal Colleges, professional bodies, and their nominees; children's charities and their nominees; survivor organisations and their nominees; voluntary and independent sector organisations providing sexual violence or domestic violence and abuse services for victims/survivors or perpetrators, and their nominees; the police, through the Association of Chief Police Officers (ACPO) leads on topics covered by the programme; National Institute for Mental Health in England (NIMHE) experts by experience network. All invited constituencies were represented in the responses received in each of the three rounds. Responses were accepted from individuals or organisations. Respondents were invited to provide responses in relation to each of the programme areas in which they considered they had expertise. There were 285 responses in Round 1, 130 responses in Round 2 and 91 responses in Round 3. Of the respondents, 68 responded in all three rounds; 23 responded to Rounds 1 and 3; 62 responded in Rounds 1 and 2 and 132 responded only in Round 1. The response rates in Round 2 and Round 3 were 46 per cent and 32 per cent respectively. Overall, 54 per cent of the Round 1 respondents replied to at least one further round (i.e. in Round 2 and/or Round 3).

Violence and abuse care pathways mapping

There were two separate strands of this work. The first looked at severe and chronic victimisation and revictimisation and covered all VVAPP areas and groups with a particular focus on learning-disabled people, physically disabled people, black and minority ethnic issues, and also organised paedo-phile and ritual abuse. The findings of this research will be published by the Survivors Trust during 2010. The second strand focused on West Yorkshire Asian women and mapped pathways to and through the many agencies with which these victims and survivors had contact; Chapter 7.2 presents find-ings from the West Yorkshire study. Case studies from previously published sources are also used to illustrate the experience of victims, survivors and perpetrators.

Methodological and other challenges

Sexual and domestic abuse and violence exists in ALL populations, regard-less of culture, religion, socio-economic status and other socio-demographic factors. Accurate estimation of its patterning in terms of relative differences in rates of occurrence is extremely difficult given a wide range of definitional and methodological challenges to estimation – including those consequent on the stigmatised and stigmatising nature of much of this violence and abuse. This issue is explored in some detail in Marianne Hester's chapter on gender and sexuality in relation to gender differences in patterns of violence and abuse.

Overview of the book

One important starting point for this book is the research carried out as part of the VVAPP programme of research and policy development. The VVAPP programme drew to a close in 2008; in producing this book, research litera-ture produced since the close of the VVAPP programme has also been included. The book's unique contribution is characterised by two features. The first of these is its scope – all groups across all areas including victims, survivors and abusers, children, adolescents and adults. The second feature is the scale, sophistication and triangulation of its research methodologies. A major contribution of this book is its use of the life-course as the analyti-cal framework for reporting on this research.

Taking a life-course approach, the book explores what is known about appropriate treatment responses to those who have experienced, and those who perpetrate violence and abuse. Part II contains four chapters. The first of these, Chapter 2, introduces the theoretical basis for understanding vio-lence and abuse, followed by an exploration of some of the overall findings from the Delphi expert study about principles, values and core beliefs, about guidelines for practice, a public health approach to prevention, and key features of an integrated approach to service provision. This sets the scene for looking in more detail at the different stages in the life-course, which follows in Chapters 3, 4 and 5. Chapter 3 covers children (taken here to include up to age 12), Chapter 4 covers adolescents and young people, and finally in Part II, Chapter 5 covers adults.

Specially commissioned chapters within the third part of the book examine key factors that are important in understanding how and why different groups experience heightened risks of violence and abuse, and the factors important in shaping appropriate responses to the particular needs of these groups. These chapters examine: gender and sexuality, race and culture; disability; and, abuse by professionals.

In Chapter 6 Marianne Hester examines the gendering of interpersonal violence and abuse; and the implications of sexuality for the experience of interpersonal violence and abuse by heterosexual, lesbian and gay individuals. While the literature on violence and abuse often considers gender and sexuality as separate issues and phenomena, processes of gendering and issues related to sexuality are by no means discrete, and Chapter 6 explores some of the overlaps, links and implications of difference. Gender is of crucial importance to understanding the impact of interpersonal violence and abuse on individuals, and understanding what may work in overcoming victimisation. At the same time, sexuality creates different experiences and outcomes. The social construction of masculinity, as embodied in heterosexual men, helps to explain, for instance, domestic violence as the exertion of power and control by men over women in intimate relationships within contexts of gender inequality (Itzin 2000b, 2000c; Hester, 2004). In same-sex relationships gender is not as prominent in positioning individuals within relationships and in interactions and constructions of power and violence. There is, however, still evidence of gendered norms impacting on experiences and outcomes of violence and abuse for lesbians and gay men (Hester and Donovan, 2009). This is explored alongside the discussion of gender throughout Chapter 6.

Chapter 7 then turns to issues of race and culture. There are two contributions within this chapter. Chapter 7.1 by Hannana Siddiqui and Meena Patel, draws on the work of, and the Department of Health-funded research carried out by, Southall Black Sisters (SBS), an organisation that, over its 30 years life, has worked locally and nationally on domestic violence, suicide and harmful cultural practices such as forced marriage and honour crimes, and related issues of racism, poverty, homelessness and immigration matters. Focusing specifically on South Asian women, the chapter argues that social cohesion, multi-faithism, old style multiculturalism or cultural relativism and racist or discriminatory policies and practices do not protect black and minority ethnic (BME) women from domestic violence or help them overcome trauma, suicide and self-harm. Policies and practices based on mature multiculturalism, secularism, equalities and human rights are the only guarantors of BME women's freedom from domestic violence and associated mental illness.

Chapter 7.2, by Jalna Hanmer, summarises findings of research on the experience of a sample of women of South Asian origin living in the North of England. The findings demonstrate how responding to domestic violence against women is extremely demanding, placing organisational demands upon agencies as well as demands for good practice on individual workers. For successful intervention, individual workers require knowledge of domestic violence, an in-depth understanding of specific women's problems and the social context in which the woman is located, the remits and abilities of other local agencies, previous agency contacts and interventions with women, and the totality of which agencies need to be involved. This demands effective multi-agency communication and collaboration.

Chapter 8 on violence, abuse and disabled people has three contributions. Chapter 8.1 by Richard Curen and Valerie Sinason focuses on learning disability. This explores the interrelationships between abuse and disability, considering the abuse experienced by those who are learning disabled, abuse by the learning disabled in parental roles as well as sex offenders. They examine and consider the need for and value of psychotherapy to the learning disabled. They identify how, although progress is occurring, much still remains to be done to ensure that learning-disabled people achieve equal access to therapeutic and other services.

Chapter 8.2 by Jackie Barron and Nicola Harwin focuses on physically disabled women. Drawing in particular on the Women's Aid study of disabled women and domestic violence, they explore how not only disabled women experience more abuse than non-disabled women throughout their lives from childhood onwards, but also how disability and abuse interact and compound each other, increasing and widening the abuser's power and control, and at the same time making it much harder for the victims to seek help. They argue that an appropriate response is to embed the needs of abused disabled women at both operational and management levels in all organisations, and in particular within those in the specialist disability and domestic violence sectors, and consider how recent policy developments may make this more difficult to achieve.

Chapter 8.3, by Ruth Marchant, focuses on disabled children. She explores the health and mental health effects of the abuse of disabled children by presenting the stories of three different children and young people and reflecting on the impact of childhood impairment and disabling barriers on their experiences. The three stories untangle some of the risk factors for disabled children, explore the strong association between childhood maltreatment and childhood impairment and consider the additional barriers faced by disabled children in getting help and accessing support. The chapter concludes by summarising the legislation and guidance that provide the current framework for safeguarding disabled children in the UK and giving practical pointers for best practice in tackling the health and mental health effects of the abuse of disabled children.

The final chapter in Part III, Chapter 9, by Sarah Barter-Godfrey, examines abuse by professionals that is, by perpetrators who are not friends or family nor strangers, but people that act in a professional capacity and through that profession come into contact with their victims. Abuse by professionals harms the social fabric and the uneven distribution of power allocated to professions, in particular their capacity to cover up misconduct, and can lead to a severe undoing of the social contract. Abuse is widespread across society, and the dimensions for enabling abuse have the potential to be applied to almost any institution or organisation. It is not possible in the scope of a single chapter to adequately represent all professions that may have abusers within their ranks or that fail to prevent abuses within their practices. Instead, four professional groups that have notably high rates of recognised abuse are considered: religious institutions, armed forces, health and therapeutic professionals, and prison and corrections officers. The chapter concludes by drawing together principles of abuse-promoting and abuse-preventing features of institutions and professions.

The final part of the book, Part IV, turns to consider what more needs to be done to tackle domestic and sexual violence and abuse, how to achieve greater success in preventing violence and abuse and in responding through earlier intervention to ensure consequences are minimised. The single chapter in this part, Chapter 10, summarises the major messages from the earlier parts of the book. From these conclusions it is possible to draw out the implications for improving outcomes for individuals through: policy development; service and practice improvement; and lastly the need for further research. The chapter highlights a number of important overarching and underlying principles: the importance of hope and recovery in the treatment of victims and abusers; the need to understand and address the gendered nature of domestic and sexual violence and abuse; domestic and sexual violence and abuse as everyone's responsibility – the core business of all health, mental health and other relevant services across sectors; the importance of addressing health inequalities and social exclusion and, finally, the value (and necessity) of a human rights framework in tackling domestic and sexual violence and abuse.

Part II

Violence and abuse through the life-course

2   Across the life-course

Before looking in detail at the different stages in the life-course, it is useful to say something about the theoretical basis of the understanding of violence and abuse presented in this book, as well as some overall features of its approach. In this chapter therefore the theoretical basis for understanding violence and abuse is summarised first, followed by an exploration of some of the overall findings from the Delphi expert study about principles, values and core beliefs, about guidelines for practice, a public health approach to prevention, and key features of an integrated approach to service provision.

Understanding violence and abuse

In understanding what leads some individuals to behave violently or abusively towards others it is important to recognise the complex interplay of a wide variety of individual, relationship, social, cultural and environmental factors. Figure 2.1 depicts the different levels in such an ecological model, from the individual, through the interpersonal, including family (defined by biology, adoption, choice), friends, to the community and then the societal level. This figure also shows how the operations of factors at the different levels are affected by a range of socio-demographic characteristics: age, gender, sexuality, class, religion, disability and ethnicity.

Within this multidimensional model, it is important to recognise that the operation of many factors is strongly affected by social position, defined differently in different societies by gender, ethnicity, sexuality, religion and a variety of other aspects. Given the social nature of many of these elements, it may be more appropriate to think in terms of a socio-ecological model of violence and abuse. Within this framework, however, as is discussed later, genetic and neurobiological factors play a part, although, not in any deterministic sense.

Some of the specific social factors implicated in the interactions involved are depicted in Figure 2.2, and these are considered further, in terms of the research evidence supporting them, in Chapters 3 to 5. This figure particularly depicts the gender differences in terms of some of the most likely effects

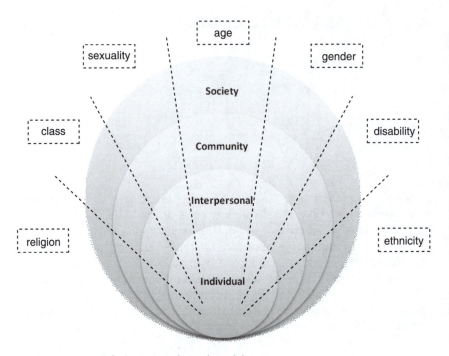

Figure 2.1 A modified socio-ecological model.

Source: original inspiration from Krug et al. (2002: 12).

produced. Once again, however, it is necessary to emphasise that the relationships shown are those of increased risk of particular proximal or distal consequences, they are not deterministic relationships. As Figure 2.2 illustrates, there are particular windows of vulnerability and opportunity, in terms of the vulnerability of the brain to damage, and the possibilities of repair.

Moving on in terms of understanding the complex interactions at work in sexual and domestic violence and abuse, Figure 2.3 summarises the major risks and impacts of violence and abuse across the life-course. The impacts cover both those in terms of mental ill-health, and through increased risk behaviours, to increased risks of negative physical health outcomes. The diagram shows the medium- and long-term sequelae of abuse experienced in childhood, and the routes through which this is associated with increased likelihood of further experience of abuse in later life, and heightened risk of multigenerational effects. The chapters following on childhood (Chapter 3) adolescence (Chapter 4) and adulthood (Chapter 5) pick up these points further in terms of the research evidence related to particular impacts.

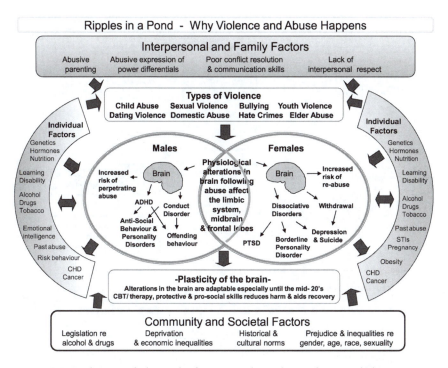

Figure 2.2 Violence and abuse: the factors implicated in violence and abuse.

Source: Nurse (2006), used with permission.

Principles, values and core beliefs

In each round of the Delphi study within the VVAPP, respondents were asked to comment on principles, values and core beliefs that should underlie practice. Analysis of the responses in Round 1 of the Delphi identified five clusters of themes that were present in the answers: power and responsibility; protection, safety and risk management; interventions; criminal justice; working together, providing and sharing information. A fair amount of commonality was identified across all 10 programme areas.

There was a strong consensus that multi-agency approaches are necessary for responding to and providing interventions for domestic and sexual violence and abuse. Sharing information between agencies is important for multi-agency work, but issues of confidentiality and data protection define and limit the sorts of information that may be shared and with whom, providing many challenges to achievement of effective multi-agency work. Public protection is an important consideration when defining the roles and responsibilities of individuals, organisations and the law. Risk assessments, both of risk to self and risk to others, are important parts of any intervention. They should be conducted by professionals, based on ethical and

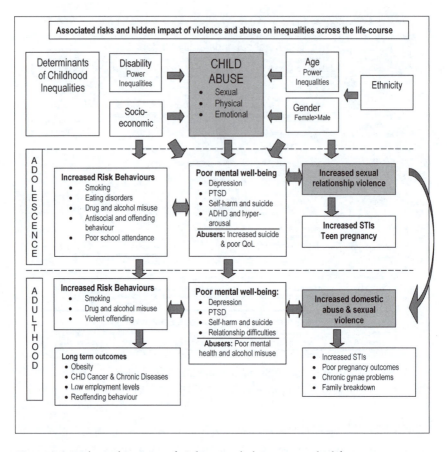

Figure 2.3 Risks and impacts of violence and abuse across the life-course.

Source: adapted from Nurse (2006), used with permission.

informed understandings of risk and potential for harm. Where appropriate, risk assessments should be carried out over time rather than as a static, single event.

For adult groups, clear differences were identified in the way victims/survivors were viewed compared to abusers/perpetrators, with responses emphasising the importance of affirming a lack of blame or responsibility for those who experience abuse: 'for victims/survivors we need to remove the guilt and responsibility so many of them wrongly attribute to themselves'. Alongside this is the need for abusers/perpetrators to accept responsibility for their actions and appreciate that they had the opportunity to act differently: 'Sexual and domestic violence and abuse are the personal choice and responsibility of the perpetrator. Other factors may play a part, but do not remove this responsibility'. For younger age groups, positions espoused emphasised a different view; for the group of children and young people who display sexually inappropriate behaviour or who sexually abuse other young people, children or adults, the following statement emerged: 'Children and young people who abuse others are not offenders, but inappropriate (and they are also seen as victims themselves)', while for young people who perpetrate domestic violence and abuse, the espoused position was: 'Young people who perpetrate DV are offenders. However, rather than criminalising them for life, they may be seen as troubled rather than pathologised.'

Tensions were apparent in the responses in relation to a number of issues:

- confidentiality versus safety and child/victim protection;
- whether full healing/recovery for victims/survivors is always possible, this may be explainable in terms of the difficulty of defining what this means; it is also linked closely to the support of openness and honesty in the course of the therapeutic relationship, while being mindful of the need to identify the most appropriate ways of working with victims/survivors in the course of the therapeutic relationship;
- whether behaviour change for perpetrators/abusers is always possible;
- the extent to which punishment and penalties act as deterrents against perpetration;
- the extent to which rehabilitation of perpetrators is essential for prevention of future offending;
- the situations in which mandatory reporting should be required.

Diversity, inclusion, equal treatment and basic human rights principles were strongly suggested as fundamentally important, suggesting that a human rights/equalities framework was a required basis for policy and practice, with explicit attention to gender, sexuality, ethnicity, and disability within this. A second overarching theme was the notion of the importance of a victim/survivor-centred approach (associated with characteristics such as empowerment, giving control and choice to victims/survivors); this was suggested, by some, to include choice for victims/survivors in terms of the gender, sexuality and age of the person they work with.

Guidelines for practice

Two sets of practice guidelines, BACP Ethical Framework (BACP 2006) and the Respect Guidelines (Respect 2004) were mentioned frequently in the responses to Round 1 of the Delphi study. The BACP ethical framework, which includes guidelines for practice, was suggested as relevant in responses from the six programme areas that deal with victims/survivors, while the Respect guidelines were suggested as being suitable for accrediting services provided in relation to services for perpetrators of domestic violence and abuse. In later rounds, respondents were asked to comment on these existing sets of guidelines. The respondents were generally supportive of both, with high percentages agreeing that they are the most appropriate guidelines presently available (Round 2; 72 per cent and 81 per cent of respondents respectively).

The Respect guidelines are very specific in relating to men's perpetrator programmes and associated women's services only (as stated in the introduction). The introduction goes on to state: 'however, many of the principles and standards will also be of relevance to those working with same-sex domestic violence, female perpetrators and family violence'. Many of the comments from the Delphi experts expressed the view that considerable modification, or even a total re-write, was required for these other contexts of work.

In addition, other respondents made reference to the desirability for adherence to suitable/relevant professional standards; there was no attempt to include all of these in detail for comment within the Delphi. Specific sets of practice guidelines that were mentioned were:

- Health Professions Council practice and ethics guidelines, see http://www.hpc-uk.org/aboutregistration/standards/;
- British Association of Social Work Code of Ethics, see http://www.basw.co.uk/Default.aspx?tabid=64;
- General Social Care Council Code of Practice, see http://www.gscc.org.uk/codes/.

Throughout the responses in the three rounds of the Delphi, views were expressed about the importance of clear guidelines/codes of ethics and practice; however, there was no agreement as to whether these should be profession-specific and/or specific to violence and abuse, or even to different types of violence and abuse. Some respondents called for specific guidelines in relation to different groups such as BME communities. Some respondents raised the concern that treating abuse as a separate case (through separate guidelines) could have the effect of isolating the sufferers even more than they are already, arguing that part of the healing is about normalising and not treating abuse as somehow different from all other life experiences. Another important point was the need to ensure that those receiving therapeutic interventions have knowledge of the relevant guidelines; as one survivor commented, in relation to the BACP guidelines: 'as a client I did not realise just what guidelines were in place but having read the report I can state that if they were consistently adhered to they would be acceptable'. Many respondents noted the importance of systems for monitoring/assuring adherence to guidelines/codes of ethics and practice (something that was not explored in detail in the study). A number of respondents noted that all sets of guidelines require regular re-examination. Since the Delphi study, the BACP ethics framework has been revised twice and the Respect guidelines once. The latest version of the BACP ethics framework is available for download from http://www.bacp.co.uk/ethical_framework/ (accessed

1 February 2010). The Respect Accreditation Standard is the document against which all member organisations will be assessed for accreditation. Many national governmental and non-governmental organisations have signed up to support this Standard, including the Home Office, Children and Family Court Advisory and Support Service (CAFCASS), the Ministry of Justice, Women's Aid, the Association of Directors of Children's Services and Relate. The full list is included with the latest version of the Standard (June 2008), which can be downloaded from http://www.respect.uk.net/ pages/principles-and-standards.html (accessed 1 February 2010).

A public health approach to prevention

As highlighted in Chapter 1, the Department of Health's Public Health White Paper *Choosing Health – Making healthy choices easier* (DH 2004b) included a cross-government strategy for tackling the root causes of physical and mental ill-health in child abuse and domestic violence, stating that:

> Child physical, emotional or sexual abuse and neglect and domestic violence are causal factors in the mental and physical ill health of children, adolescents and adults and affect a significant proportion throughout their lives. The high costs in prevalence and economic burden on health and social care services and criminal justice system have pushed these issues up the agenda.
>
> (p. 41)

The Public Health delivery plan *Delivering Choosing Health: Making healthier choices easier* (DH 2005c) included joint Department of Health and Home Office action to develop Sexual Assault Referral Centres (SARCs) nationally, including services for children and adolescents. It also included targeted action to improve the quality of patient experience through the joint Department of Health, Home Office and National Institute for Mental Health in England violence and abuse programme.

The Delphi experts overwhelmingly emphasised the importance of a public health approach to prevention, first and foremost aimed at changing societal attitudes to violence and abuse. In the later chapters of the book, the elements of this approach are described and related to the research evidence that underpins them; in this chapter the elements of the approach are briefly outlined below.

Sexual and domestic violence and abuse need to be made public health issues, with a public awareness campaign stressing personal responsibilities and rights; much more openness and acknowledgement of levels of sexual violence and abuse is needed. There needs to be an engagement with the media to ensure a balance between airing the sensational or confrontational aspects of abuse (which attracts good audiences) and the important but softer informational and educational content that those who are quietly or secretly living with memories prior to disclosure need. Awareness and information sessions need to be provided in schools as part of the Personal, Social and Health Education curriculum. Sexual and domestic violence and abuse need to be made priority issues for education services, with additional support for teachers who are supporting pupils who disclose.

The need for application of a basic public health model (of identifying risk factors and strengthening protective factors in the individual, the family, the community and society within various age bands) was emphasised. Prevention needs to be approached as any other major public health campaign, with appropriate components for primary, secondary and tertiary prevention:

- Primary prevention – work in all sectors (schools, youth settings, workplaces) aimed at changing attitudes to all forms of violence and abuse. Large-scale public awareness programmes aimed at changing attitudes to violence and abuse, to include understanding of what consent means, need to be carried out at general population level and within all cultural/ethnic communities involving women in the community and community leaders. Stronger sanctions against perpetrators. Perpetrator-focused media campaigns. Work within particular groups upholding practices that are violent and abusive; examples include forced marriage, female genital mutilation and gang cultures supportive of rape and abuse of women.
- Secondary prevention – better risk assessment. Effective interventions by criminal justice system to hold perpetrators to account. Specialist prosecutors. Better targeting of those that are vulnerable to abuse or being abused including service provision, helplines, support work, etc. and engaging adults in abuse prevention. Training and building skill capacity within a wide range of statutory and voluntary agency workers in order to begin to address the problem when it does present itself to services. Early identification and intervention with families (to be carried out in a range of different settings, e.g. GPs, mental health, maternity, A & E departments, social services, schools). Appropriate systems (information sharing and intervention protocols) in place to ensure early intervention in any abuse of their clients by professionals.
- Tertiary prevention – therapeutic support for survivors, effective treatment and accountability for perpetrators. One very important aspect is to make it easier to report crimes and reassure victims about how they will be supported.

Children and young people are most likely to be safe and kept safe if they understand their right to be safe, have been helped to develop the confidence to speak out if they feel danger, or do not like what is happening; have a secure base within family or substitute family; and there is at least one adult they can talk to. Therefore building children's self-esteem and self-worth, and listening to and taking them seriously should be at the core of all universal services and should be part of a strategy in, say, PHSE for equipping children to grow safely and healthily, with an understanding of healthy relationships and consent. This needs to be developed through adolescence into knowledge and understanding about safe dating. Education of learning-disabled people about sexual activity and relationships is also required.

Throughout all sectors of society, organisations need to proactively 'model' non-abusive and empowering behaviours. Workplace bullying and harassment policies have a role to play here.

A less punitive and more therapeutic approach is required towards the perpetrators, who must be treated firmly and appropriately and not let off or cautioned. Adequate resources to be able to offer and to require the uptake of treatment must be available as there is evidence that these can work in the case of domestic violence perpetrators as illustrated by the case study EP. There must be zero tolerance of violent and abusive behaviour for a programme to be effective.

Case study EP: DV perpetrator in receipt of effective services

EP was physically bullied at school and abandoned by his father at age 6, for example describing an incident where his father came to his house when he was younger but hadn't identified himself. He had a stepfather who he described as a highly supportive and 'real' father. His relationship of over ten years had a long history of violence; at one point, his wife had sought refuge but her daughter convinced them both to try again. Prior to his entry onto a perpetrator programme (15 weeks of CBT and role play) his reported violence to his wife was occurring weekly.

At the time of interview, months after the end of his programme attendance, he had been violence-free for three to four months, something of which he was proud, but he further identified that he was still financially and verbally abusive. He also conveyed that he was embedded in his own process of reaching towards non-abusiveness. He spoke with consistent and deep empathy about his wife, and although he had stopped his violence he openly admitted and described his other abuses that he was still working on eliminating. He ascribed switching jobs to one closer to home and with a better overall environment as an important part of his ability to behave better towards his wife. He spoke highly and often of the programme facilitators, expressing gratitude for the challenges offered by them that led to his change. In his own words:

... I didn't want the group to end.
We did a lot of role playing, but the main one, were when me

and XXX paired up, and I were XXX's daughter, and obviously XXX were XXX. We played that out, how he'd treat her, and I'd be XXX, and he'd be the daughter, and we played that out. And when I were being XXX, I were stood over him, XXX ... started crying. And then obviously we did it, I were wife, XXX were me, and we did it that way round. And that, I think that, were one of the main things in group, actually. Made you feel how your partner was feeling. You know, with XXX, he had me standing over him, he wouldn't have had that, and he probably hadn't all in his life. And the first time he's realised what his girl-friend must have felt. Same for me. I had XXX standing over me, 16, 17 stone lad, waving his finger, shouting abuse, and you think, that's what my wife went through, you know? So, that's the one thing, you never want to drop that out of group. Really brings it home, it does. So a lot of the stuff were subtle, going in there, but that one, it was such an impact.

(From Garfield, S. (2007), used with permission)

Other important components of service provision include an increase in the availability of advice to those who know they have a sexual interest in children, such as confidential free phone numbers and a need to have facilities available for those who have no criminal record but who are concerned about their behaviour/desires. Also relevant here are restrictions on availability of pornographic material, given the role of such material in increased risk of developing pro-rape attitudes, beliefs and behaviours, and committing sexual offences (Itzin et al. 2007).

One issue on which diverging views were apparent was whether domestic violence/abuse and sexual violence/abuse should be separated for prevention work or not. This can perhaps be resolved if primary prevention is distinguished from secondary and tertiary prevention. For primary prevention, programmes benefit from targeting all forms of violence and abuse (and indeed it is hard to separate them for such work), whereas when secondary and tertiary prevention are considered, approaches benefit from being more specifically targeted.

Key messages and key challenges – across the life-course

The first and foremost point to emphasise is the possibility of healing and prevention from violence and abuse. This is not to offer any simple guarantees in terms of 'magic bullets' that can be formulaically applied. Instead, responding to the needs of those who experience and perpetrate violence and abuse is a creative art and science, utilising a variety of approaches – an essentially human and relational process:

It was a chance remark, by a therapist colleague, about those who had experienced CSA as being "too damaged to recover, beyond hope" that caused me the most intense distress, yes sure, that was the fear I'd battled against for years, but, at those times when I connect with the reality of the successes of my life I know it is not true. It seems to me that for professionals to casually undermine that knowledge is outrageous, instead they should be holding up the knowledge that healing is possible to help us progress in our own recovery.

(Personal communication from CSA survivor, used with permission)

Although knowledge is not complete (as chapters throughout the book will emphasise), enough is known to clearly set out what needs to be done and how to achieve it. This is not to say, however, that making the required changes will be easy. A number of major challenges remain. First and foremost is the necessary political will to support, and to resource, the services and policy initiatives required.

As the book demonstrates, changes are necessary throughout all sectors of society in order to achieve the necessary whole of system/society implementation to address violence and abuse adequately. Political will is necessary, not just in the short term, but into the medium and long term, as the necessary changes and implementation of a public health prevention framework cannot be achieved in the short lifetimes of single governments.

A major component in what is necessary is effective interagency collaboration, based on clear understanding of the complementary roles that different agencies have to play within an overall public health framework, and clear protocols to permit information and resource sharing.

Success will not be complete, however, without breaking through the silence and shame that still cloaks much violence and abuse; silence and shame on behalf of the victims or survivors who fear condemnation and blame from those individuals and agencies who should provide support and services, and silence and shame on behalf of perpetrators who wish to hide their responsibility for their acts and actions and refuse the possibility of change. This requires a major change in attitudes in society, moving away from a view that sees violence and abuse as perpetrated by the evil stranger to views that see violence and abuse as something that needs to be tackled throughout the fabric of society, in private as well as public spheres. As the foundation for this change, recognition of the centrality of human rights, and respect for diversity and difference, are essential to addressing the needs of both victims/survivors and perpetrators.

3 Violence and abuse through the life-course

The importance of childhood

Children ... do not have the wherewithal to give informed consent to engage in sexual activity with adults. The responsibility for abuse always lies with its perpetrator. Sexually abusive behaviour in adults is not an illness but is chosen behaviour. The confidentiality and civil liberties of adults who abuse children must give way to the rights of children to be safeguarded from harm. Children can recover from child sexual abuse. Recovery will be substantially assisted if at least one adult they know and trust believes them and sticks with them. Because of the enormity of the violation that child sexual abuse inflicts on a child – in that it distorts their sense of self and distorts or interrupts their development – most children will need some help from someone to recover from its impact. Building resilience in children and young people will assist them to recover and assist safeguard from being further targeted and abused. The needs of the criminal justice system (an adult arena where sanction is considered and meted out principally on behalf of society as a whole) should not take precedence over the needs of children to recover from their experiences and develop strategies for future safety. The vast majority of children who are abused will be targeted by someone they have some kind of emotional attachment to – therefore understanding how best to assist them will need to take account of and have understanding of their 'groomed environment' – what/who has stopped them speaking out. Children who tell will have made a decision at some level that it is better to tell than not tell – they will usually have weighed up that telling will feel 'least worst'. There are more subtle issues around communication when children tell through their behaviour/functioning.

(Delphi expert, CSA)

Understanding how best to act in preventing and responding to violence and abuse directed against children remains one of the most difficult challenges facing societies today. The subject is fraught with denial, with stigma, with shame, and with heightened emotion. While public and media attention is often directed against abuse perpetrated by strangers, the sad reality is that the majority of abuse in childhood is perpetrated by those known to the child – by parents, relatives, family friends (Itzin 2000a, 2002; May-Chahal and Cawson 2005). Confronting this unpalatable truth, that abuse against children is predominantly perpetrated by those within relationships of trust, still requires further development in our understanding as to how best to educate, intervene and respond in ways that support the healing of all those involved. Stranger danger, however, also deserves careful attention, particularly in the context of the ever increasing availability of the internet within homes to those of young ages.

This chapter is concerned with children who have been sexually abused, with child victims/survivors of sexual exploitation in prostitution, pornography and trafficking, with child victims of domestic violence and with children who display sexually inappropriate behaviour. Child neglect, physical violence and emotional/psychological abuse against children are not covered in detail within the chapter – although it is important to acknowledge that one or more of these is or are often found alongside sexual abuse, domestic violence, and sexual exploitation.

In this chapter the nature and extent of domestic and sexual violence and abuse in childhood are first summarised and then the effects of domestic and sexual violence and abuse in childhood and beyond examined, before looking at the behavioural impacts of abuse, at coping strategies and resiliency. The fourth major section discusses children's expectations of health and social care sectors and considers what is known about what children want from service providers. The chapter then moves on to discuss the service response, first in terms of prevention, then in terms of responding to children who display sexually inappropriate behaviour, and then in terms of psychological therapies and other therapeutic interventions.

The nature and extent of domestic and sexual violence and abuse in childhood

Chapter 1 reviewed the difficulties in establishing accurate figures about numbers of new or continuing cases of sexual violence and abuse. Studies present a wide range of different statistics and it is impossible to conclusively establish the reasons for the differences. Pereda and colleagues (2009) reviewed studies of the prevalence of child sexual abuse, updating the review of Finkelhor (1994). They found among 39 studies carried out in 21 countries, giving similarly wide ranges of prevalence estimates for women and men (0 per cent to 53 per cent and 0 per cent to 60 per cent respectively), the highest rates for both men and women were from a study in South Africa. The range of estimates is wider than that found in Finkelhor's earlier study.

Within the UK, the NSPCC undertook a national prevalence study of child maltreatment and found that 21 per cent of women and 7 per cent of men reported sexual abuse as a child (Cawson et al. 2000). Gallagher and colleagues (2008) report findings from a school-based questionnaire survey of sexual abuse and abduction occurring outside the home; children included were aged 9 to 16. The reported prevalence rate for at least one attempted or completed incident of CSA or abduction was 21.9 per cent. For those reporting at least one incident, a stranger was the perpetrator of the last incident in 34.9 per cent of cases, and a non-stranger in 50.8 per cent; data was missing in 14.3 per cent of cases. A study by NCH Action for Children found that 75 per cent of mothers reported their children had witnessed domestic violence, 33 per cent had seen their mothers being beaten and 10 per cent had witnessed sexual violence (Abrahams 1994).

Studies of learning-disabled children and youth that included comparisons to non-disabled children and youth (Sullivan and Knutson 2000; Verdugo et al. 1995) found that maltreatment was 3.1 to 7.66 times more prevalent among learning-disabled individuals. Kvam (2004), reporting a Norwegian study, finds the hearing-impaired are more likely to be abused. Horner-Johnson and Drum (2006) reviewed the literature on maltreatment of learning-disabled children, finding that this indicated that they may be particularly at risk of sexual abuse.

Social, cultural, and economic factors contribute to child sexual exploitation through gender bias, discrimination, poor education, and poverty (Willis and Levy 2002). Risks of sexual exploitation (Chase and Statham 2005; Taylor and Quayle 2003) rise with:

- Experience of abuse and disadvantage;
- Experience of being a 'looked after child'/ in care;
- Disrupted family life;
- Problematic parenting;
- Disengagement from education (truancy and exclusion);
- Substance misuse;
- Poor health and well-being, low self-esteem;
- Being physically or learning disabled.

Effects of domestic and sexual violence and abuse, in childhood and beyond

> Do you want to know how I feel about it? It gets me all confused and muddled up. When it happens I feel as if things are growing in my head, outwards and pressing on my head. Do you want me to give you an example? I'll tell you what, I'll tell you a good example, but you'll have to have lots of paper to write it down! There was a big argument one day. My dad didn't want his tea. He bought me an ice cream. He punched her three times. Someone came running out. He kept kicking her. Mum was crying and crying. And then I got mad – I'm not a nasty person, really I'm not, but I just got mad. Then he kicked his car. Then he got in it and then he got out again, and he came for me so I ran away. Later, I played with my sister on the computer. My mum was being looked after by our neighbour. Then we saw the police and I went to my

auntie's. Have you understood it? It just gets me so muddled up. I'm frightened I'll be like it when I grow up. I know what she is going through and I want to help her. I get worried for her.

(8-year-old mixed race boy on his experience of
domestic violence, quoted in Mullender et al. 2002: 95–6)

Impacts of domestic and sexual violence and abuse on children are immediate, widespread and long-lasting. In an analysis of American data from the National Comorbidity Study, Zielinski (2009) finds evidence to suggest that those who experience child maltreatment are at increased risk for financial and employment-related difficulties in adulthood. A multigenerational study identifies an increased risk of negative health and other effects for the children of women who were sexually abused as children (Noll et al. 2009). Many of the systematic reviews in existence do not consistently distinguish between different age groups, and many are concerned with identifying medium- and long-term effects of childhood abuse in later life as an adolescent or adult. Neigh and colleagues' review (2009) on the neurobiological effects of child abuse and neglect summarises the pervasive and long-term effects as shown in Table 3.1. A summary of key recent literature from reviews and individual studies is given in Table 3.2; this draws on reviews carried out by the authors and the recent reviews of evidence carried out as part of the process of production of the recent NICE guidelines on child maltreatment (NCCWCH 2009).

A helpful review of the impact of exposure to domestic violence on children is provided by Holt and colleagues (2008), illustrating the increased risk of abuse, emotional and behavioural problems and of adversities, such as parental substance abuse, insecure housing, parental mental health issues, that follow from exposure to domestic violence; note, however, that this review is descriptive rather than critical or systematic. Jenny and colleagues (2008), discussing child abuse, emphasise that complex traumatic stress suffered early in life has both behavioural and developmental consequences. The brain's physiological adaptations to the abnormal world of child abuse,

Table 3.1 Pervasive and long-term effects of experiencing child abuse and neglect

---

- Neurodevelopmental Delays
- Hypothalamic–pituitary–adrenal (HPA) Axis Dysfunction – the HPA axis is a major mediating pathway of the stress response
- Metabolic Syndrome – combination of medical disorders that increase the risk of developing cardiovascular disease and diabetes
- Cardiovascular Disease
- Immune System Dysfunction
- Major Depressive Disorder
- Post-Traumatic Stress Disorder
- Compromised Reproductive Health
- Transgenerational Effects

Source: drawn from Neigh et al. (2009: 392).

Table 3.2 Effects of experiencing domestic and sexual violence and abuse in childhood

	Sources
Delayed/reduced development and poor educational attainment	Carlson (2000) Dixon et al. (2006) Edleson (1999a) Kitzmann et al. (2003) Paolucci et al. (2001) Veltman and Browne (2001)
Poorer physical health and injuries	Kemp et al. (2008) Sox (2004)
Antisocial and offending behaviour	Dixon et al. (2006) Edleson (1999a) Evans et al. (2008) Sox (2004) Wolfe et al. (2003)
Sleep disorders	Wells et al. (1995)
Anxiety and psychological problems	Evans et al. (2008) Kendall-Tackett et al. (1993) Kitzmann et al. (2003) Valente (2005) Wolfe et al. (2003)
Eating disorders	Smolak and Murnen (2002) Wonderlich et al. (2000)
Depression and PTSD	Evans et al. (2008) Glaser (2000) Kendall-Tackett et al. (1993) Luthra et al. (2009) Paolucci et al. (2001) Valente (2005)
Self-harm, suicidality and suicide	Evans et al. (2004) Paolucci et al. (2001) Valente (2005)
Dissociative disorders	Collin-Vezina and Hebert (2005) Glaser (2000) Kisiel and Lyons (2001) Lansford et al. (2002) Macfie et al. (2001)
ADHD and hyper-arousal	Glaser (2000)

although initially useful, become problematic in the world outside the abusive home.

The behavioural impacts of abuse

The guidelines produced for the National Institute for Health and Clinical Excellence (NCCWCH 2009) provide a useful summary of behaviour that should lead to consideration or suspicion of child maltreatment; see Table 3.3.

Table 3.3 Guidelines for suspicion of child maltreatment: emotional, behavioural, interpersonal and social functioning

---

Behavioural disorders or abnormalities either seen or heard about

---

- **Disturbances in eating and feeding behaviour**

Suspect child maltreatment if a child repeatedly scavenges, steals, hoards or hides food with no medical explanation.

- **Sexualised behaviour**

Suspect child maltreatment, and in particular sexual abuse, if a prepubertal child displays or is reported to display repeated or coercive sexualised behaviours or preoccupation (for example, sexual talk associated with knowledge, drawing genitalia, emulating sexual activity with another child).

Suspect past or current child maltreatment if a child or young person's sexual behaviour is indiscriminate, precocious or coercive.

Suspect sexual abuse if a prepubertal child displays or is reported to display unusual sexualised behaviours. Examples include:
- oral–genital contact with another child or a doll
- requesting to be touched in the genital area
- inserting or attempting to insert an object, finger or penis into another child's vagina or anus.

- **Self-harm**

Consider past or current child maltreatment, particularly sexual, physical or emotional abuse, if a child or young person is deliberately self-harming. Self-harm includes cutting, scratching, picking, biting or tearing skin to cause injury, pulling out hair or eyelashes and deliberately taking prescribed or non-prescribed drugs at higher than therapeutic doses.

- **Wetting and soiling**

Consider child maltreatment if a child has secondary day- or night-time wetting that persists despite adequate assessment and management unless there is a medical explanation (for example, urinary tract infection) or clearly identified stressful situation that is not part of maltreatment (for example, bereavement, parental separation).

Consider child maltreatment if a child is reported to be deliberately wetting.

Consider child maltreatment if a child shows encopresis (repeatedly defecating a normal stool in an inappropriate place) or repeated, deliberate smearing of faeces.

- **Runaway behaviour**

Consider child maltreatment if a child or young person has run away from home or care, or is living in alternative accommodation without the full agreement of their parents or carers.

Emotional and behavioural states

Consider child maltreatment if a child or young person displays or is reported to display a marked change in behaviour or emotional state (see examples below) that is a departure from what would be expected for their age and developmental stage and is not explained by a known stressful situation that is not part of child maltreatment (for example, bereavement or parental separation) or medical cause. Examples include:
- recurrent nightmares containing similar themes
- extreme distress

Note:
'consider' child maltreatment means that maltreatment is a possible explanation for a particular feature.
'suspect' child maltreatment means a serious concern about the possibility of child maltreatment but not proof of it.

(Continued)

Table 3.3 Continued

Emotional and behavioural states

- markedly oppositional behaviour
- withdrawal of communication
- becoming withdrawn.

Consider child maltreatment if a child's behaviour or emotional state is not consistent with their age and developmental stage or cannot be explained by medical causes, neurodevelopmental disorders (for example, attention deficit hyperactivity disorder (ADHD), autism spectrum disorders) or other stressful situation that is not part of child maltreatment (for example, bereavement or parental separation). Examples of behaviour or emotional states that may fit this description include:

- Emotional states:
  - fearful, withdrawn, low self-esteem
- Behaviour:
  - aggressive, oppositional
  - habitual body rocking
- Interpersonal behaviours:
  - indiscriminate contact or affection seeking
  - over-friendliness to strangers including healthcare professionals
  - excessive clinginess
  - persistently resorting to gaining attention
  - demonstrating excessively 'good' behaviour to prevent parental or carer disapproval
  - failing to seek or accept appropriate comfort or affection from an appropriate person when significantly distressed
  - coercive controlling behaviour towards parents or carers
  - very young children showing excessive comforting behaviours when witnessing parental or carer distress.

Consider child maltreatment if a child shows repeated, extreme or sustained emotional responses that are out of proportion to a situation and are not expected for the child's age or developmental stage or explained by a medical cause, neurodevelopmental disorder (for example, ADHD, autism spectrum disorders) or bipolar disorder and the effects of any known past maltreatment have been explored. Examples of these emotional responses include:

- anger or frustration expressed as a temper tantrum in a school-aged child
- frequent rages at minor provocation
- distress expressed as inconsolable crying.

Consider child maltreatment if a child shows dissociation (transient episodes of detachment that are outside the child's control and that are distinguished from daydreaming, seizures or deliberate avoidance of interaction) that is not explained by a known traumatic event unrelated to maltreatment.

Consider child maltreatment if a child or young person regularly has responsibilities that interfere with essential normal daily activities (for example, school attendance).

Consider child maltreatment if a child responds to a health examination or assessment in an unusual, unexpected or developmentally inappropriate way (for example, extreme passivity, resistance or refusal).

Source: produced from, NCCWCH 2009: 11-13© Royal College of Obstetricians and Gynaecologists; reproduced with permission.

Note:
'consider' child maltreatment means that maltreatment is a possible explanation for a particular feature.
'suspect' child maltreatment means a serious concern about the possibility of child maltreatment but not proof of it.

The guidance makes a careful distinction between two levels of concern: to 'consider' child maltreatment means that maltreatment is a possible explanation for a particular feature whereas to 'suspect' child maltreatment means a serious concern about the possibility of child maltreatment but not proof of it. The guidance also uses the terms 'unsuitable explanation' to mean an explanation that is implausible, inadequate or inconsistent with other features. For pre-pubertal children, child maltreatment, and in particular sexual abuse, is associated with repeated or coercive sexualised behaviours or preoccupation (NCCWCH 2009; Putnam 2003).

All forms of child abuse and neglect occur within a context of relative powerlessness of the child and lack of control over what happens to them. Since abusive behaviour to the child is often unpredictable, unconnected to the child's behaviour, and interspersed with declarations and/or acts of affection, the lack of predictability, uncertainty and lack of control combine to create circumstances in which children adopt a variety of strategies, which, although allowing the child to gain a sense of control, are all too often seen as signs of pathology rather than a coping mechanism (Godsi 2004; Jenny et al. 2008). This lays the basis for a wide range of problems in later life.

Experience of abuse and/or neglect during development is particularly serious owing to its impact on the process of development itself, increasing the risk of psychiatric and other medical disorders above those associated with exposure to abuse in adult life. The process of brain development in children is constantly modified by environmental influences, and, for the young infant, the primary caregiver(s) exert(s) considerable influence over the environment. Abuse and neglect have distinct but interacting effects on development (Glaser 2000), through the different ways that they can affect brain functioning. Many of these effects are related to aspects of the stress response, through alterations to the hypothalamic–pituitary–adrenal (HPA) axis, and have consequences in terms of hyper-arousal, aggressive responses, dissociative reactions as well as educational underachievement. It is, however, extremely important to recognise that not all children exposed to abuse and/ or neglect demonstrate altered HPA axis physiology. Neigh and colleagues' review (2009) summarises the importance of considering genetic influences on outcomes from exposure to child abuse and neglect, identifying that not enough is yet known about the genetic variables which, in combination with particular clusters of environmental factors, confer risk or resilience on particular individuals. Intergenerational effects of abuse, both in terms of physical and mental consequences, are also identified within Neigh and colleagues' review (2009). Although there is evidence indicating sex differences in the acute neuroendocrine stress response, the current information is insufficient to draw conclusions about the specificity of the neuroendocrine system in explaining female–male differences in acute trauma responses (Olff et al. 2007). A meta-analysis to examine the relationship between childhood exposure to domestic violence and children's internalising, externalising, and trauma symptoms (Evans et al. 2008) showed that the relationship between exposure to domestic violence and externalising symptoms was significantly stronger for boys than for girls.

Case study RP: Childhood sexual abuse – incest and paedophilia in one perpetrator

RP experienced quite a lot of physical violence as a child. The physical abuse was very visible in the family, but it was interpreted in a particular way (i.e. she was naughty, rude, ill-mannered) so it could be accommodated. Her father deliberately injured her with her mother present, but her mother claims at that time she didn't realise what he was doing was criminal. RP said she viewed her mother's decision to be inactive with quite a lot of cynicism: that for her mother maintaining the nice middle class happy family image was far more important than what was actually going on. Her father was careful not to mark her where it would be very visible.

Her first memories of sexual abuse were when she was a toddler. As a young child there was a lot of digital penetration. Her mother said from a very early age she was waking after having a recurrent nightmare about a nasty big bad scary man who was horrible and just like a monster and he had a big stick in his hand and he would chase her with it and stab her and it was red on the end. She couldn't work out how her mother could say she knew nothing. She didn't like what he was doing and was very frightened of him when he was doing those things, but the rest of the time she said he was her dad and she basically loved him. From the age of seven to 15 the sexual abuse got worse.

She made many disclosures that were ignored, to social services who took down her address and never followed up. She went to the family doctor on three occasions with a friend from school. He asked her when it was most sore between her legs, meaning her vagina, and she said 'it hurts most when something big gets taken out like my dad's fingers or his penis'. The doctor was a family friend who went to the same church as her mother. By the time she got home he'd phoned her mother and she knew she was in big trouble.

She was referred to a Child and Adolescent Psychiatric Unit, but each time she went with her parents and they stayed with her for the entire duration of the discussion, and she couldn't talk openly in front of her parents. When she was 15 she told her mother that her father had been sexually abusing her and her mother said she believed her but there wasn't anything we could do.

When she was seventeen her parents started divorce proceedings. She was anxious to prevent her father having unsupervised access to her younger brother and sister and wrote a letter to the court, but the

Crown Prosecution Service dropped the case and her father got full unsupervised access. However, about five years later, the police contacted her for a statement because they knew of another child who had been abused by her father. He ended up being charged and found guilty of four offences and sentenced to 14 years. She said 'We've got a conviction now and that's very good, but he had seven additional years to abuse as many children as he wanted'.

(Source: summarised from chapter 6 in Itzin (2000))

In terms of exposure to sexual and domestic abuse, children's diverse responses have been explained by theoretical frameworks including social learning, stress and coping, trauma, and risk and resilience. While many argue that social learning theory best explains behavioural effects such as aggressive behaviour, other theories are more able to account for other effects. Not all children are equally adversely affected by exposure, as case study RP illustrates, so an understanding of protective and other factors which may moderate or increase risk (e.g. severity of violence, frequency and duration of exposure, and maternal coping strategies) is important for framing appropriate responses (Carlson 2000; Kolbo et al. 1996). The concept of resilience, understood, not as some form of innate toughness inherent in only a few individuals, but a human capacity that can be developed and strengthened in all people, through relationships, specifically through growth-fostering relationships (Hartling 2008), is useful in understanding the differential patterns of response that can be observed in situations of violence and abuse.

One of the most disturbing things for me was the realisation in later life of how my mother had constructed a view of the world as a highly dangerous place, conveying this vividly to myself and my siblings, in order to justify to herself not trying to change anything that was going on within the home – after all – it is safer than anywhere else ... that view of the world as a dangerous place was one that held me back and took me years to unlearn.

(Personal communication from CSA survivor, used with permission)

In the literature on coping strategies it is common to distinguish between two different types: avoidance and approach (Roth and Cohen 1986). Avoidance coping is seen as a passive strategy, it involves denial, behavioural disengagement, distraction, and sometimes withdrawal or hiding, whereas approach or problem-focused coping is seen as active coping, involving planning, positive reframing. A subset of this involves seeking support (emotional or instrumental). A further type of coping distinguished is venting coping, involving venting and self-blame. Avoidance coping is often labelled as maladaptive, and while this may be an accurate description in the long term, in the short term, for a young child, this may be the best, or even only, available strategy. The advisability of labelling particular types of coping as maladaptive is to be questioned in any case, as it runs the risk of undermining victims' acts of resistance in the face of abuse, and mitigates against the facilitation and support of strengths-based approaches to coping.

Some abused children exhibit resilience despite the severe adversity in their lives (Cicchetti and Rogosch 1997; McGloin and Widom 2001), as case study RP illustrates. Unfortunately not enough is known about how such resilience can be facilitated and supported. Research into protective and supportive factors is limited, but has already identified three general categories of important protective factors: individual; family; and external support systems (Hartman et al. 2009). A recent study by Schultz and colleagues (2009) found three potential protective factors, social competence, adaptive functioning skills and peer relationships, were positively related to outcomes for children investigated for maltreatment. Research is also beginning to illustrate the range of social and cultural factors that can play a protective role. For example, Kim (2008) demonstrates that child religiosity may largely contribute to a stress-coping process among children from low-income families; his study also indicates that the protective roles of religiosity varied by risk status and gender. One problem, however, is that the scope of operation of such protective factors, particularly within the individual and the family may be compromised by the abuse, or its consequences, for example in having to re-locate to escape domestic violence: 'Leaving everything behind is hard – my real dad, my brothers, my sisters, my cousins, my whole family really … we had to leave the town that I've lived in for ten years' (10-year-old girl quoted in Humphreys and Thiara 2002: 32).

Exposure to violence and abuse in childhood is of particular importance given its scope for enhancing the likelihood of negative effects in later stages of life. This occurs not only through what the child learns about acceptable behaviour and responses to different situations, but is also linked to neuro-biological effects mediated by genetic and environmental factors as discussed earlier. While attention is often paid to the vicious cycle of abuse, and to intergenerational effects, it is important to emphasise that most of those who are victims of abuse in their own childhood do not go on to abuse others (Langstrom 2001).

Behavioural responses such as such as hyper-vigilance or extreme passivity, can be useful, even life-saving coping responses to an abusive home; they are less useful when they are present in a non-threatening environment, and all too easily are labelled as pathology and responded to in ways which do not assist in the development of different behavioural responses for the non-abusive environment, but rather reinforce the problematic behaviour (Jenny et al. 2008). As Jenny et al. (2008) emphasise, non-abusive caregivers for a child with difficult behaviours need to understand the roots of these behaviours and to learn ways of responding to these.

Expectations of health and social care sectors: what do children want from service providers?

Within the Delphi study, owing to the ways that experts were recruited, it can be assumed with confidence that none of the experts by experience were children aged 12 or less at the time of the Delphi study. This section is therefore based in research studies in the literature that have interviewed children aged 12 or less about their experience of abuse, including child sexual abuse and domestic violence. One problem is that many studies work with a wider age group and do not separately identify those aged 12 or less. Three of the exceptions in the domestic violence research literature are UK studies carried out by McGee (2000a, 2000b), Mullender et al. (2002) and Humphreys and Thiara (2002). All the studies emphasise the children's knowledge and understanding of the domestic violence within the family and illustrate the wide range of coping strategies that the children drew on to survive the situation, as well as to intervene to try and protect their abused parent. This was true of children under 12 as well as the older children. The children gave very clear messages about what they wanted from service providing agencies.

They wanted to be talked to, to be allowed and encouraged to express their opinions and to be involved in decisions (by non-abusing parent, by agencies, including the police, by service providers, in refuges etc.). Children talked about wanting to be given information about what is going on, and about service options and availability. They valued opportunities to talk to other children in similar situations. A key expectation from services was provision of safety, for themselves and the abused parent; this was also expressed in terms of a call for the provision of more refuges, including provision of refuges for specific groups: 'The people at the refuge helped us the most. They did this by making our life happier, by taking us out. They made us feel better by taking everything out of our minds as if it didn't happen' (9 year old South Asian girl, quoted in Mullender et al. 2002: 101)

Although there is a large body of research with children who have experienced CSA, very little of the research focuses directly on the child's experience of services. From the literature from adult survivors, some clear conclusions emerge. First of all, is the need to be believed and taken seriously, and to have disclosure reacted to in a sensitive and caring fashion, with no attribution of blame to the child. Second is the need for safety, for action that removes the possibility of further abuse, and enables the child to feel safe. It is also important for children to have a voice in decisions and about service provision, even at a very young age, children can express their preferences and wishes.

A key issue is disclosure and the recognition that there may be huge obstacles for children to do this. They may have been threatened by the abuser and live in fear of anyone finding out. There is often shame and self-blame. They may worry that a disclosure would break up the family and they may be put in care. Very young children may not have the words to describe what has been happening to them. Based on the sample of children identified in Cleveland in 1987, Bacon and Richardson (2000) provided a detailed explanation of the psychological factors that influence disclosure; in older children subject to prolonged abuse and trapped in silence, or those for whom there is a high index of suspicion, medical evidence may be the one opportunity for them to break the silence.

What forms of prevention work?

The first aspect to emphasise is the importance of primary prevention, universal programmes aimed at whole populations – to tackle cultures of normalised violence and sexualisation of children, to give knowledge of rights to choice and control to children, and to empower them with the skills and confidence to assert their own wishes. Society-wide programmes aimed at adults are dealt with in Chapter 5. Here programmes targeted at children are considered, focusing first on programmes in schools and then on programmes outside schools.

Primary prevention: programmes in schools

A variety of programmes cover school based social development training and student education and skill development regarding abuse awareness and prevention, anti-bullying, 'healthy' relationships (family and friends), and seeking help. Topping and Barron (2009) report a systematic and critical review of the efficacy of purely school based child sexual abuse prevention programmes. They searched the literature published between 1990 until 2005, and identified 22 studies for inclusion, the latest of the included studies were published in 2001. Studies did not have to have a comparison group, but did have to include outcome measurement. Key outcomes included personal safety knowledge, self protection skills, emotional impact, perception of risk, changes in disclosures, maintenance of gains and negative programme effects. Over the 14 studies for which an effect size could be calculated, the mean effect size was 0.61 – a moderate effect size. Negative effects were reported in half the studies, these were mostly small in number, mild in nature and of short duration. The authors report poor quality in many studies, acknowledge the difficulties of research in this field and conclude that the positive results reported in the better quality studies provide some encouragement – but are not sufficient to warrant whole-hearted endorsement of the programmes without further research. They identify guidelines from examining the programmes with larger effect sizes and four or more outcome gains – concluding that modelling, discussion and skills rehearsal are crucial programme components, and that programmes should also be at least 4–5 sessions long, have the capacity to be delivered by a range of personnel and involve active parental input.

There is also some evidence supporting whole school approaches for behaviour improvement, including bullying and abuse prevention: with staff training on educational and communication styles; prevention policies, including improved nutrition and physical exercise (NICE 2008). There are potential roles in delivering these for a wide range of public sector professionals (for example health visitors, school staff or police) as well as the voluntary and community sector. Complementary to programmes aimed at children are those aimed at parents in terms of parent education programmes, fostering development of warmth, positive regard, empathy, the use of clear and consistent boundaries and positive discipline (NICE 2008); these are considered further in Chapter 5.

Primary prevention: programmes outside school

Most out of school prevention programmes target at risk children or families. One exception is described by Dubowitz et al. (2009), who report encouraging results from an RCT of a primary care based preventive programme that produced significantly lower rates of child maltreatment on a number of measures, but more extensive evaluation is required.

Programmes targeted at high risk groups include: home visiting programmes; pre-school enrichment programmes; protective skill training for abuse prevention for children at high-risk for abuse, (e.g. looked after children, disabled children, families experiencing domestic violence); training of professionals in contact with children in order to identify abused children to refer for protection, therapy and protective skill training; early identification of abusive behaviour, for example, conduct disorder, in children for additional pro-social skills and parenting programme interventions.

Hahn et al.'s (2003) systematic review concludes that there is sufficient evidence of the effectiveness of early childhood home visiting in reducing child maltreatment (physical, sexual, or emotional abuse; physical, emotional, or educational neglect; or a combination of abuse and neglect) in families at risk for maltreatment, including disadvantaged populations and families with low-birthweight infants. MacMillan with the Canadian Task Force's (2000) review reaches similar conclusions (although expressed somewhat more cautiously), and a later review by Gonzalez and MacMillan (2008) clarifies that while most programmes targeting at-risk families have not shown evidence of effectiveness in preventing abuse or neglect, there were two exceptions, the Nurse Family Partnership and the Early Start programme (see Table 3.4).

According to Macmillan et al. (2000), evidence remains inconclusive on the effectiveness of a comprehensive health care programme, a parent education and support programme, or a combination of services in preventing child maltreatment. Sure Start local programmes, designed to improve the health and wellbeing of children living in disadvantaged neighbourhoods do not directly target abuse, but they do contain factors known to be protective or promotive of resilience, among their outcome variables. Some encouraging results have emerged from the evaluation of the fully established Sure

Table 3.4 Successfully targeting at-risk families

	Nurse Family Partnership	Early Start programme
Country	United States	New Zealand
Provided by	Nurses	Nurses and social workers
Provided to	First time socially disadvantaged mothers	Family with 2 or more risk factors
Beginning	Prenatal, before end of second trimester	Postnatal, before 3 months after birth
Programme length	During pregnancy and 2 years after birth	As soon after birth as possible until child aged 3
Programme intensity	Visits weekly for first four weeks, then fortnightly for remainder of pregnancy. Weekly for first six weeks after birth, then fortnightly until child aged 21 months, then monthly until age 2 years	Dependent on family need
Programme activities	1. Promoting healthy pregnancy, health and development of child and parent's life course 2. Assisting women in building relationships 3. Linking women and family with health and social services	Comprehensive assessment of family needs, resources and strengths, followed by collaborative generation of solutions to family challenges (partnership between home visitor and client)
Evaluation follow-up	Over 15 years	Over 3 years
Outcomes compared to control group	• Improvements in women's prenatal health behaviours and pregnancy outcomes • Children – higher intellectual functioning, lower behavioural problems, less emotional vulnerability and language delays • Rates of child abuse and neglect reduced in first two years postpartum for highest risk women • Fewer deaths aged 0–9 from preventable causes • Reduction in maltreatment at 15 year follow up (not at 4 years) • Presence of intimate partner abuse reduced programme effects on maltreatment, but not on maternal or child functioning	• Children had greater contact with primary health care (doctors and dentists) and less likely to have hospital visits for injury or ingestion • Higher rates of positive and non-punitive parenting at 36 months • Lower rates of severe child assaults • No differences in family related outcomes including maternal health, family functioning, exposure to stressful life events, economic circumstances

Source: summarised from Gonzalez and Macmillan 2008.

Start programme (Melhuish et al. 2008) in terms of positive effects on five out of fourteen outcomes: children's social development; children's social behaviour; children's independence; less negative parenting; and better home learning environment. Melhuish et al. (2007) analyse the data further to examine whether variations in the programmes account for the differences in child/family functioning, and find modest links between implementation characteristics, including empowerment of parents, and effectiveness for child and parenting outcomes. This provides helpful information to guide future programme design.

The VVAPP systematic literature review could identify no studies that examined the efficacy of screening for child abuse. MacMillan et al.'s (2000) review of literature on the prevention of child maltreatment found that screening approaches used to identify families at high risk for child maltreatment generated high false-positive rates and high risk of mislabelling people as potential child abusers. Parental education and support programmes led to a decreased number of reports of child abuse and neglect. Programmes aimed primarily at preventing sexual abuse of children, by increasing awareness and improving safety skills, have been shown to improve children's knowledge of sexual abuse and enhance their awareness. However, none of the studies examined actually determined the effectiveness of programmes in reducing the incidence of sexual abuse or abduction.

Failure to provide appropriate interventions for children who experience violence and abuse in childhood (including witnessing domestic abuse) lays the ground for increased risk of problems in later life, increased likelihood of further experience of abuse for female children and increased likelihood of abusive behaviour for male children. It is important to stress here, however, that what is at stake is increased risk rather than inevitable fate. Not all girls who are abused go on to become abused women and not all boys who are abused go on to become abusers. The clear inference from this is that appropriate intervention can be tailored to minimise adverse consequences, and, the experiences of children who have been abused have important messages to yield about the factors and circumstances that assist recovery and reduce the risk of further abuse experiences as either victim or perpetrator. Particularly important in this is the presence of positive experiences, for example at least some constant, consistent relationships of support/affection/love/positive regard from adults. This may be from a family member, family friend, health or social care professional, school teacher, etc. (Godsi 2004). Societal attitudes and expectations about gender roles are also important, and Chapter 6 considers this further.

Secondary prevention: working with children who display sexually inappropriate behaviour

The research that exists (Hackett 2004; Whittle, Bailey and Kurz 2006), as well as expert opinion, supports the adoption of broad-based behavioural and developmental goals, with the use of a cognitive behavioural framework, and attention to the resolution of the child's own abuse experiences. Work that includes the non-abusing parent is also supported. Interventions that are supportive and empathic, and tailored to the developmental stage of the child are important; these need to pay careful attention to the child's unique constellation of experiences that have shaped their presenting behaviour.

The most common position advanced by the Delphi experts was that appropriate intervention required long-term engagement and an holistic approach to working with both the individual child and their carers/family, an eclectic or multi-model approach was strongly supported. It was strongly emphasised that all work needs to be contextualised within the family/care system in which the child lives, and careful preparation, including extensive assessment and risk planning is necessary before long term therapeutic interventions:

> With children who sexually abuse other children, working both on their own victimisation if they have been abused but not shrinking from working on their abusing behaviour and ensuring that those around them (e.g. caregivers in substitute care or parents) do not minimise and deny this behaviour.
>
> (Delphi expert)

> A multi-agency, systemic approach to case management; Rigorous, evidence based assessment; A range of measurable treatment interventions drawing on theoretical models including Cognitive behavioural therapy (CBT), Multisystemic Therapy (MST) and psychodynamic principles; One size does not fit all with children showing sexually harmful behaviour since they have diverse needs. A diversity of evidence-based treatments will need to be designed to meet these needs.
>
> (Delphi expert)

Attention was particularly drawn to the need to recognise learning disability in formulating treatment strategies, and the importance of relating planned interventions to stage of development.

Except for zero-tolerance, all of the specific therapeutic approaches named in the Delphi questionnaire were reported as useful/helpful by some of the Delphi experts (Appendix 3). A strongly supported position was that provision of residential options was important for some children/young people (not however within the context of offender institutions).

There were a number of tensions in the responses: the extent to which a cycle of abuse should be regarded as inevitable or not and the extent to which early intervention in this is possible; whether touch/holding has a place within therapeutic approaches or not. Other positions within the Delphi that emerged were: that there are insufficient interventions for abusing children; drop-out is the single factor that most compromises the effectiveness of intervention; the engagement of the young person in the management of his/her problems is crucial.

Supporting healing: psychological therapies and other therapeutic interventions

> Although love and consistency are essential, they are not always enough.
> (Jenny et al. 2008: 668)

Within the Delphi study, there was a strongly supported view on the victim/ survivor side that therapy choice should depend on both the individual and the context, and that the quality of the therapeutic relationship is particularly important. Connected to this was strong support for the use of integrated or mixed approaches, the view that there is no single approach that is best for everyone, and that different approaches each have their place in a staged process of intervention (without, however, implying simple sequential ordering in this process). Integration also applies in terms of the need to integrate therapeutic and treatment interventions with other services that may be required. A wide range of particular approaches were viewed as helpful for children by the experts by both profession and experience who participated in the Delphi study; see Appendix 3. Therapeutic approaches should support and build on protective factors including relationships with carers, friendship networks and educational opportunities. The next three subsections deal with specific findings for: children who have been sexually abused; children who are victims of domestic violence and abuse; children who have experienced commercial sexual exploitation.

Children who have been sexually abused

For children who have been sexually abused, the strongest position emerging from Delphi experts was on the value of interventions structured around a victim-centred approach, using age, gender and developmentally appropriate techniques:

> Different interventions work for different children. If very young, non-directive play therapy has proved beneficial, if older a more holistic approach involving cognitive and other intervention approaches. Most of all young people and children need to make sense of what has happened to them, understand where the blame lies and be empowered.
> (Delphi expert)

> Narrative therapy can be used in play therapy as a way of helping children express and explore their experiences of life. Every story a child tells contributes to a self-portrait which he can look at, refer to, think

about and change, and this portrait can be used by others to develop an understanding of the storyteller. The stories we tell, whether they are about real or imagined events, convey our experience, our ideas, and a dimension of who we are. The therapist and child construct a space and a relationship together where the child can develop a personal and social identity by finding stories to tell about the self and the lived world of that self. The partnership agreement between child and therapist gives meaning to the play as it happens. The stories created in this playing space may not be 'true' but often will be genuine and powerfully felt and expressed.

(Delphi expert)

The human qualities of the therapeutic relationship were emphasised as very important, as was the need to work with the non-abusing parents, carers, siblings and others in the child/young person's network. The importance of therapists understanding and being able to work with dissociation and dissociative disorders was emphasised. In providing therapeutic interventions, the importance of an understanding of lesbian, gay and bisexual development and affirmation for sexuality was stressed.

For some of the specific therapeutic approaches listed in the Delphi questionnaire (CBT, feminist/pro-feminist, mediation/alternative dispute resolution, family systems, mutual support/self-help, restorative justice, relapse prevention), at least one of the experts raised some concerns in answer to the question about what approaches should not be used and why. Most of the points raised related to the use of particular approaches being unhelpful at particular points/stages, or in particular circumstances, rather than the approach being totally counter-indicated. For example, some experts drew attention to the range of therapies recommended as suitable prior to a criminal trial in Crown Prosecution Service guidance (CPS 2001), which excludes hypnotherapy, drama therapy, regression techniques and groups in which disclosure of assault details takes place. Other experts were concerned about the application of particular techniques owing to the danger of re-traumatisation (visualisation, blank screen technique in psychoanalysis, re-living exercises). For some, behavioural and cognitive approaches can be characterised as too superficial without 'healing' type interventions, in other words were viewed as only being able to be a part of the interventions required, and it was stressed that they must be implemented in a developmentally appropriate fashion.

There were a number of areas in which incompatible positions were evident and no consensus was achieved at the end of the Delphi process. The first of these was whether touch/holding has a place within therapeutic approaches. The Delphi responses contained many comments on the use of touch in therapy, these illustrated the complexity of the issues to be considered, including the nature of the therapy (the difference between massage therapy and counselling for example), and the importance of a distinction between touch and holding. While survivor choice and wishes were seen by many as providing a governing principle, others identified the danger of clients consenting 'to keep a therapist happy', and the difficulty of understanding this for young children.

A second area of lack of consensus was whether it is ever appropriate to have a therapist of the same gender as the perpetrator. A possible resolution of this would be through adoption of the position, also advanced, that victims/survivors should be offered choice in this area, another option is the use of pairs of therapists. In later Delphi rounds, all the experts agreed that choice of therapist was ideal, however many noted that it was not always, or even often or ever, possible to offer this. A number of experts reiterated that the more important factor was the quality of the relationship created with the therapist rather than the therapist's gender. Experts noted the importance of recognising that children may have experienced abuse by females or by both males and females:

> Therapeutic groups for children (and parents/carers) which are for same gender and similar developmental stage, which are structured and time-limited, and which have a psycho-educational approach can be helpful in some ways. Children tend to associate these groups with school 'lessons' and this fact, along with meeting other children with similar experiences, can really help reduce stigmatisation, the sense of being different, and loneliness. Also, as a male working with female co-therapists, I have found these groups can also provide a different experience of a male and model an effective parental couple. In general, groups with children need to be conducted alongside parallel work with parents/carers to ensure that therapeutic benefits are supported and sustained. Although groups cannot reach some areas of distress, as a positive therapeutic experience, they can help some young people move on to individual therapy.
>
> (Delphi expert)

There were also tensions around the difficulty of establishing the appropriate point for therapeutic intervention to start. While an ideal position was that of establishing safety first, all recognised that this situation rarely came about quickly. Some expressed the view that safety should be established first and that it was potentially harmful for therapeutic intervention to start if abuse is ongoing. Some cited the difficulty or even impossibility of ensuring no further abuse, arguing that it is harmful to delay the start of therapy. Some distinguished different types of therapeutic support for different circumstances. Quotes from two different Delphi experts illustrate the tensions graphically:

> The idea that therapy is withheld in cases of ongoing abuse seems to me to be akin to a firefighter refusing to switch on a hose to put out a

burning house until the people in the house have left. What is required of a therapist at the stage of ongoing abuse is a different set of skills than when the person is safe, but it is unethical and unprofessional to abdicate responsibility when the client remains in danger.

(Delphi expert)

The mental health of the survivor is unlikely to be improved whilst the trauma is ongoing. I often say to clients that if their house was on fire, a fireman is far more useful in the short term than a psychologist!

(Delphi expert)

There were also some tensions about the extent to which joint work with family is possible and desirable, while there was a strongly supported position about working with supportive elements in the child/young person's network, the question of accurately distinguishing supportive elements is obviously relevant here. A recent meta-analysis of parent-involved treatment for CSA (Corcoran and Pillai 2008), which included seven studies (five of which were provided by a single research team, leading the review authors to sound a note of caution since overlap (or lack of it) in the different studies' populations was not ascertainable) provided evidence that (non-abusing) parent-involved treatment does provide some advantage over comparison treatments (typically child-only treatment), over four domains: internalising symptoms, externalising symptoms, sexualised behaviours and PTSD.

Comments made in all rounds of the Delphi in relation to therapeutic approaches for children who have been sexually abused emphasised particularly the complexity of the issues involved, the need for flexibility, and for facilitating control and choice by the individual client:

In my own experience I believe in working alongside the survivor, I see them as the expert, in as much as they know their limitations and with help and support the worker and survivor can plan a suitable pathway to dealing with their issues. In my opinion it is vital the survivor stays in control of the therapeutic relationship. Survivors need a worker who will stay with them, be consistent, open and honest in their approach.

(Delphi expert)

Absence of the strongest forms of evidence about positive effects from different therapeutic models is not however the same as evidence of the absence of any positive effects. Instead it reflects a lack of relevant research and of rigorous research of high quality. The limited literature available from systematic reviews and meta-analyses is highly consistent with the findings from the Delphi experts. Hetzell-Riggin et al.'s (2007) systematic review examined interventions for sexually abused children, here authors' concluded the best approach would be client specific which focused on secondary conditions. Macdonald et al.'s (2006) Cochrane review examined studies of cognitive behavioural interventions for children and adolescents who had experienced child sexual abuse, finding evidence in support of cognitive behavioural treatments. In slight contrast Ramchandani and Jones' (2003) systematic review found evidence to support the use of cognitive behavioural interventions for sexually abused children of pre-school age, though its efficacy for older children was less clear. They also report that involving the non abusive parents was found to be beneficial for the child. Reviews by Cohen and colleagues (2006) and Saunders and colleagues (2004) each identified evidence for a wide range of different therapeutic modalities; Cohen and colleagues in particular also suggest existing models could be adapted for additional types of traumas, developmental levels, co-morbid conditions and levels of severity and chronicity, mirroring the views expressed by the Delhi experts. In terms of options for early intervention, Glaser's (2000) review of the effects of child abuse and neglect on the brain, suggests that acting on factors that support resiliency, enhance self-esteem and encourage self-organisation (within the older child) are particularly important, as is the construction of a coherent account by the child of her or his own experiences (Glaser, 2000).

The majority of studies and reviews have focused on CBT approaches to treating sexually abused children. To fill a gap in the evidence base, exacerbated by the absence of RCTs in this area, as part of the VVAPP the Department of Health commissioned guidelines on *Psychoanalytic Psychotherapy after Child Abuse* about the treatment of adults and children who have experienced sexual abuse, violence and neglect in childhood (McQueen et al. 2008). This was produced by a guideline development group comprising all of the relevant professional and training bodies together involving the Children's charities as well as clinicians, and the Survivors Trust representing adult survivors of childhood sexual abuse. It focuses on psychoanalytic treatments for children (and adults) who have been sexually abused and covers the nature and extent of the problem, its contexts, symptoms and effects in childhood, including children with disabilities, socially excluded children, child abuse linked to spiritual or religious belief, trafficked children, online abuse and adolescents and children who commit child sexual abuse, with discussion of attachment, trauma, dissociation and the developing brain.

Children who are victims of domestic violence and abuse

For child victims of domestic violence and abuse, victimisation and autonomy of the client are comparatively diffused, and three considerations emerge: the role of the child in a household affected by domestic abuse; the role of the non-abusing parent; and, the role of the abusing parent. The overarching position held by the Delphi experts was that there should be no assumptions made about the type of therapeutic interventions that are needed by children and adolescent victims of domestic violence and abuse, instead, service provision should be predominantly needs led, guided by the age and maturation of the child and their individual experiences and degree of victimisation.

The child's position in a household where there is domestic abuse was recognised as ambiguous; they may be a primary or secondary victim, through direct experience or through witnessing acts of DV; they may have experienced persistent, sporadic or isolated DV incidents; they may have experienced DV from a number of household members, in series or from only one person; and, they may or may not have suffered from the compounding effects of the various potential mental health outcomes for the non-abusing parent. For some Delphi experts it was possible to view children as 'witnesses', but for other Delphi experts it was important to emphasise children as social actors within the DV household, that had their own behavioural contribution to maintaining their own safety and developing coping strategies.

From this ambiguity, the Delphi experts advanced two competing, but not necessarily incompatible, approaches to therapeutic interventions for children and adolescents with regard to the role of the non-abusing parent. First, the position that children should have access to information, confidentiality and legal help in their own right and make their own contribution to decisions made about their lives and therapies; note here the similarity in position to that discussed earlier in the section on what children want. Second, the position that the child's relationship with the non-abusing parent should be preserved, and its enhancement should be seen as an aim of therapeutic interventions, and indeed also note here that this position is reflected in the views from the children discussed earlier. In this second position, taken on its own, it becomes harder to separate the child as an autonomous figure in the therapeutic process, though there is an assumption that mutually acceptable decisions can be reached where there is a preference, or need, to be treated separately.

As with children who had experienced sexual abuse, some of the Delphi experts considered, that, although the ideal position might be to ensure the safety of the child before starting therapy, the possibility of ensuring safety in the short term is often limited, and the distinction between 'support' and 'therapy' hard to define unambiguously. Other experts however expressed a forcefully argued position that safety and separation are prerequisites to therapies:

> Child protection issues and safety of a placement must be resolved before any ongoing therapeutic treatment is practicable and ethically acceptable; there can be pressure from the professional network for therapy to start a.s.a.p. and before the former has been resolved adequately.
>
> (Delphi expert)

Alongside the position that therapies can only be undertaken after the child is assured to be in a safe environment (usually through safe separation of the non-abusing parent from the DV perpetrator), there is a position that recognises the ongoing role that a DV abusive parent may take in the child's life, and subsequently that the DV abusive parent may also play a role in family therapies:

> If the perpetrator is able to remain part of the family safely (as in some cases of domestic violence), then family therapy can help in the delineation of responsibility in the family and the acknowledgement of the effects of past events.
>
> (Delphi expert)

In contrast, some Delphi experts saw involvement of the abusing parent (usually the father) as problematic:

> Need to challenge the myth of 'any contact with fathers is worthwhile' that still informs major decisions over child contact with abusive men, even in the presence of 'evidence' to the contrary.
>
> (Delphi expert)

One Delphi expert by experience highlighted the problem of involving the DV perpetrator in forms of family therapy when he is also (unknown to the mother or the therapist) sexually abusing his children, and how this can have a silencing effect on those children which becomes enforced and entrenched by the power his involvement in family therapy bestows upon him.

In relation to safety and separation, a number of experts emphasised the need for consideration of these separately. Some argued that safety was the more important, and that separation was not as important. The dangers of separation were also noted, and the complexity of the issues involved:

> The need for safety is paramount but separation is more complex. We must recognise the harm done to children by leaving them with abusing parents and must guard against being too naïve when assessing potential for change in an appropriate timescale for any child. Children may need support from outside the family during any period of upheaval but formal therapy may be more effective once major decisions have been made like where the child will live and who will have contact.
>
> (Delphi expert)

All of the therapeutic approaches listed in the Delphi questionnaire were reported useful/helpful by some Delphi experts (see Appendix 3). Some experts were critical of any approaches that involved contact between the perpetrator/abuser and the child (mediation, restorative justice) and raised concerns about maintaining the safety of the child. Also some experts discussed PTSD and trauma work as too severe for younger children who do not have the emotional or cognitive ability to process and engage in trauma-focused techniques.

Due to the heterogeneity of this programme area by age, extent and impact of victimisation, most experts emphasised the need for assessment prior to intervention, both of the child's needs and their maturation and developmental abilities to engage meaningfully in therapies. As well as a general position that different children are suited to different interventions, experts emphasised that specific interventions may be appropriate for different age groups: younger children are better suited to play therapies and older children may benefit from more cognitive and psycho-educational approaches.

There were thus two key areas in which consensus was not reached: (i) whether it is acceptable for the DV perpetrator and child to be included within the same programme of therapy and whether children should be engaged in family therapy where there is a history of DV; and (ii) whether it is beneficial for the child's therapeutic intervention and pace to be considered as independent from or inherently connected to the non-abusing parent's therapy.

Turning to the evidence from systematic reviews, Feder and colleagues (2009) included a review of interventions with children who had experienced domestic violence where there was also involvement of the mothers. The review was limited to quantitative studies meeting stringent quality criteria, resulting in analysis of seven papers reporting five studies. The results were promising in terms of outcomes for children and their mothers. However it should be noted that the majority of the interventions were with women who had left the abusive relationship and so the results may not be generalisable to those remaining with the abusive partner.

Children who have experienced sexual exploitation

The strongest position emerging from the Delphi experts for this area was on the value of intervention and service provision structured around a victim-centred and multi-agency staged approach. Responses stressed the importance of ensuring safety as the first stage in any intervention and the need to stop the abuse/exploitation, prior to moving on and healing through the application of any therapeutic intervention. Trauma symptoms needed to be alleviated before relational aspects were dealt with. One important issue was the need to build sufficient trust in order to facilitate sufficient disclosure in order to understand what problems need to be therapeutically addressed, and the quality of the human contact involved in any intervention was identified as important. The importance of including a focus on skills and personal development, and improvement in self-esteem were stressed. Characteristics of the overall approach are summarised in Table 3.5. The importance of therapists understanding and being able to work with dissociation and dissociative disorders was emphasised.

There are important differences between working with those 'at risk' and those leaving or experiencing direct exploitation. There are also important differences according to the age of the victims involved: 'a more structured group work approach based around activities works with young people up

Table 3.5 Characteristics of a staged, multi-agency, victim-centred approach

---

- Respect for the child victimised by prostitution, pornography, trafficking;
- An understanding of the methods of entrapment used by sexual exploiters during the grooming process and after entry into prostitution;
- Provision of opportunities for disclosure;
- Belief that they can have and are entitled to a better quality of life;
- Give the child the time to speak of their experiences, what happened, how they felt and feel, what they would like to do to regain a better life;
- Give emotional support that conveys that they can have a better life and are worth it;
- Ensure the abuser(s) do not have access to her/him;
- Provide information and support that empowers parents and other family members so that they can offer more effective support to their daughter/other relative as they are being groomed and sexually exploited prior to and after entry into prostitution;
- Adopt a multi-faceted approach to victims, i.e. responses to drug addiction, the need for safe housing, health services, social services involvement, employment/ education.

---

to 14 years,' and 'when working with children it is important that we have a range of verbal and non-verbal interventions to suit the individual'.

Child protection requirements obviously play a key part, and there is an emphasis on the difference between those who characterise the victims as children and therefore debate child protection and consent purely in terms of immaturity to be responsible for one's actions and those who talk about adult coercion, grooming and vulnerability.

All of the specific therapeutic approaches named in the Delphi question-naire were reported as useful/helpful by some of the experts (see Appendix 3). For some of the specific therapeutic approaches listed in the questionnaire (CBT, family systems, group therapy, drama therapy), at least one of the experts raised some concerns in answer to the question about what approaches should not be used and why. Most of the points raised related to the use of particular approaches being unhelpful at particular points/stages, or in particu-lar circumstances, rather than the approach being totally counter-indicated. For example, as mentioned earlier for other groups, some experts drew atten-tion to the range of therapies recommended as suitable prior to a criminal trial in CPS guidance (CPS 2001), which excludes hypnotherapy, drama therapy, regression techniques and groups in which disclosure of assault details takes place. Other experts were concerned about the application of particular tech-niques owing to the danger of re-traumatisation (visualisation, blank screen technique in psychoanalysis, EMDR, reliving exercises).

The view that punitive approaches to the victims or those 'nearly' in prostitution, pornography or trafficking should not be used was particularly strongly expressed. One part of this critique related to the use of secure accommodation/units, another to the use of child protection procedures, and yet another to approaches that encouraged prosecution:

Secure Accommodation should not be used as a principal and reactive measure to safeguard children and young people who continue to be sexually exploited.

(Delphi expert)

[There should not be] immediate movement into the child protection procedures and reporting to police and social services, such that enquiry will take place. This is likely to: put the victim in danger; put others in danger; stop the victim accessing appropriate health care; stop the victim accessing appropriate emotional care.

(Delphi expert)

Any intervention that treats children/young people subject to sexual exploitation as criminals [should not be used]. ... Trafficked and smuggled children/young people should not be identified simply as illegal immigrants but as victims of exploitative migration.

(Delphi expert)

Conclusions: caring for children

Two adult women who experienced abuse as children, research participants in a study by Thomas and Hall (2008), reflect on their healing:

My abuse happened, yes, I don't down-play that, but I don't have to dwell on it. ... I choose to make my life happier ... If you cannot find that open door, crack and push it open. There's always a little light, you just have to stick your finger in there ... and then walk through.

('Ruth', Thomas and Hall 2008: 157)

My life is wonderful ... I have this passion to help other women ... My therapist is helping me with balance, I've always been on a roller coaster. ... and I am trying to learn to live in the middle.

('Carmen', Thomas and Hall 2008: 158)

As will be seen repeatedly through this book, while knowledge of what works, and how, and for whom is imperfect, a lot is known about what has been found helpful, and there are also some clear messages about what is not helpful. It has been noted above that there is widespread agreement between the views of the Delphi experts and that emerging from the research literature, in those areas where there is research. Some important areas where consensus was not found have also been discussed, indicating the need both for further research and for clear guidelines for practice. Responses to children who have experienced sexual abuse, assault and exploitation have been undermined by severe resource constraints, and an adequate response to their needs requires this to be addressed.

4 Across the life-course
Youth, young people and adolescence

Overview

Adolescence is a period of maturation and physical, sexual, social and life-role development. As a transition between childhood and adulthood, it is the shortest of the three life stages presented here and bridges childhood and adulthood, with the emergence of individual responsibility for the perpetration of abuses. During puberty, gender roles become more salient, and dating relationships are initiated; these shifts in social/sexual roles present new opportunities for power, control and appropriate conduct to be negotiated and therefore also opportunities for abuse, violence and inappropriate conduct to occur. Throughout the rest of this chapter, adolescents will be considered both as victims and abusers, across a spectrum of violence and sexual abuse.

The nature, extent and health effects of domestic and sexual violence and abuse in adolescence

Young people experience multiple forms of abuse and violence: from their peers now old enough and strong enough to be a physical or sexual threat, from their dating partners who may or may not also be adolescents, within their families, witnessing domestic violence and experiencing the effects of living in a violent or disrupted home, and directly from abusive parents. Adolescence is also a time of increased risk from victimisation by bullying at school, as well as 'street' violence and harassment, as young people retain a vulnerability and immature assertiveness of their own authority while moving increasingly in unsupervised and independent social settings.

In adolescence, domestic violence (DV) may diverge into two forms: family violence and dating violence. Dating violence has a prevalence of 20–46 per cent in adolescence (Whitaker et al. 2006; Shorey et al. 2008), with more incidents associated with increasing age. A critical review of estimates indicates a higher prevalence of psychological or emotional abuse, compared to physical abuse, and lower prevalence of sexual abuse than physical abuse in adolescent dating violence (Shorey et al. 2008).

Using a broad description of dating violence, which includes pushing and yelling, as well as acts of intentional injury or intimidation, demonstrates less gender disparity than in adult DV. However, sexual victimisation in adolescence is more 'traditionally' gendered, with female adolescents more likely than male adolescents to be sexually assaulted (Hickman et al. 2004). Serious IPV, including the use of weapons and causing injury or hurt, is more commonly perpetrated by young men, and more frequently attributed to being used to control their partner, compared to young women who reported their acts of IPV as being attributed to self-defence (ibid.). Both male and female adolescents attribute their acts of IPV to anger, and emotional immaturity is inferred in the causation of much low-level IPV during adolescence, something that is 'grown out of' and which dissipates in the transition to adulthood (ibid.). At the point that dating and family settings overlap, teenage parenthood, is particularly risky for incidents of DV (Silverman et al. 2004).

The experience of parental DV can be harmful for adolescents (see Chapter 5 for further discussion on the prevalence and effects of DV), and for older children an increasing understanding of DV can be conflicting; they may be pressured to keep violence concealed and therefore feel complicit or oppositional to the abused parent, or they may be pressured to engage in acts of DV, under duress and through emotional manipulation by the abusive parent/family member. Adolescents may also act out their own forms of domestic violence against their parents or siblings, particularly as expressions of underlying problems or trauma, although not necessarily caused by the family members against whom they act out violence.

Prevalence estimates for sexual abuse perpetration by adolescents are exceptionally difficult to establish. Most adult sex offenders begin their offending trajectory before the age of 18, and around a third of sex offenders in contact with the judicial system are adolescents (Lovell 2002; Reitzel and Carbonell 2006). Estimates indicate that the majority of young sex offenders are aged 11–17 and male, but over 10 per cent are younger than 10 years old and about 10 per cent are girls (Vizard et al. 2007). As young women who sexually abuse others are comparatively uncommon, services and specialised interventions for them are also uncommon (Bunting 2005). In research from the US, there is some indication that female adolescent sexual abuse perpetrators tend to be identified and arrested at a younger age than young male abusers, and that their own abuse experiences tended to have started younger (Vandiver and Teske 2006).

The majority of adolescents that engage in sexually inappropriate behaviours are not in contact with the judicial system and are not necessarily 'offenders'. Conversely, young people that are coming into contact with the criminal system are not necessarily acting in ways that are inconsistent with normal sexual development, for example, 'sexting', sending sexually explicit images of oneself through picture text messages, has conflated young people's (possibly misguided) exploration of their bodies with the production and transmission of child pornography. Therefore it is important to recognise a spectrum of inappropriate sexual behaviours, ranging from that which is age-inappropriate and unhealthy, through abusive and harmful behaviours, to that which is intentionally manipulative and victimising.

Sexual and physical victimisation are associated with a range of poor health outcomes, including physical, psychological and social sequelae both as immediate outcomes of abuse, such as injuries, and long-term health problems (Hetzel-Riggin et al. 2007; Whitaker et al. 2006; Zimmerman et al. 2006). There is an emphasis on mental health and behavioural effects experienced during adolescence. Sexually transmitted infections and poor sexual health may be indicative of sexually inappropriate conduct as well as victimisation. Victimisation during adolescence is associated with depression, sleep problems, fear and anxiety, anger and aggression, low self-esteem, and increase in suicide and parasuicide. As adolescence is a critical time of identity formation and developing sexuality, victimisation can be associated with confusion over sexual identity, and more broadly associated with conflicting emotional responses that may come from feeling attached to or love for an abuser, as well as feeling harmed, hurt, ashamed and/or fearful.

Self-harm and behaviours associated with victimisation in adolescence

Victimisation in adolescence is associated with an increase in self-destructive behaviours, including drug and alcohol misuse, physical self-harm, eating disorders, suicidality and promiscuity. Experiencing sexual abuse and/or domestic violence, especially in childhood, is associated with an early initiation of sexual relationships and an increased risk of teenage pregnancy and subsequently the health sequelae associated with that, including gynaecological problems, poor nutrition and lower socio-economic attainment (Bair-Merritt et al. 2006). The experience of sexual abuse in childhood is particularly associated with an increased risk of sexually risky behaviours in adolescence and sex-trading and forms of prostitution are over-represented in adolescence (Arriola et al. 2005). The relationship between early victimisation and teenage pregnancy may be mediated by early sexual initiation and reduced capacity for managing sexual boundaries in relationships (Blinn-Pike et al. 2002). As within the adult population, sexual abuse and domestic abuse often co-occur, and both coercion and physical violence or threats increase the incidence of adolescent pregnancies. Studies of adolescent suicide have identified child physical and sexual abuse as common predisposing factors (Evans et al. 2005).

Experiencing violence and abuse is associated with running away from home, which in turn is associated with social isolation, homelessness and poor health outcomes. Homelessness in young people is at least partly created by their lack of access to welfare and financial support independent of the family unit, and young people who separate themselves from their abusive backgrounds have lower educational attainment and less capacity for employment. Problems in school, truancy and fewer school successes are all associated with both those who are victimised and those who victimise others.

Intergenerational effects and victims who become abusers

Early sexual abuse and experience of domestic violence increases the likelihood of an individual victimising others and increases the likelihood of becoming revictimised in adolescence and adulthood (Bornstein 2005; Classen et al. 2005; Roodman and Clum 2001). This occurs broadly along gender lines: abused girls are more likely to be victimised as young or older women and abused boys are more likely to perpetrate violence and abuse as young or older men (Itzin 2000a). This may be in part the consequence of learned roles, whereby young people learn social scripts that facilitate men as aggressors and sexually dominant, and women as passive and sexually subservient. However, this is far from inevitable and the majority of adolescents who have experiences of victimisation do not go on to perpetuate a cycle of abuse. In adolescence, the content of abuse may contribute to the short-term enactment of abusive behaviours. For example, adolescents may be forced to take sides or be complicit in the abuse of a parent within a DV household, or may be 'groomed' into an abusive role. It is also important to emphasise that abusive conduct in adolescence does not necessarily perpetuate into adulthood, as evidenced by higher rates and different patterns in dating violence during teenage years compared to adult patterns of DV (Whitaker et al. 2006). In particular it is important to emphasise that, while lifetime sex offenders usually begin their offending prior to adulthood, inappropriate sexual conduct during adolescence does not necessarily lead to a sex offending trajectory.

Protective factors and resilience

Several protective factors have been identified, protecting against initiation of abuse and its long-term effects, including a supportive and stable family environment, school attainment and success, individual assertiveness, age-appropriate sex education and positive role models, both within the peer-group and as responsible adults. Surveys of young people commonly find violence-supportive attitudes, especially that hitting women and coercing sex is acceptable, and societal influences and attitudes may lead towards or away from resilience, and community education is implicated in developing resilience in young people (DH 2005b). Programmes that seek to build resilience against victimisation and perpetrator-hood in adolescent dating, including education, knowledge and attitude elements, have been identified as a 'promising approach' reducing rates of perpetration for both boys and girls compared to controls (Whitaker et al. 2008: 160). There is also some emerging evidence that adolescent boys' and girls' resiliency is built by different combinations of factors, although both genders seem to be more resilient when more protective factors are accumulated, including home and school environments and measures of self-worth (Hartman et al. 2009). For young people in foster care, resiliency also appears to be built by an accumulation of positive factors, including internal factors such as perceived self-competencies and external factors such as social support and engagement with social activities (Hass and Graydon 2009).

Risk factors and identification of adolescents at risk

Anger, family background, youth culture and traumatic experiences have all been identified as risk factors for youths at risk of perpetrating a range of violence. Young people with severe conduct problems who perpetrate violence usually locate the source of their violence in anger; girls more often emphasise anger coming from painful experiences such as bullying or trauma in their past, whereas boys more often emphasise anger originating from current obstacles and circumstances that 'require' violence (Biering 2007). Parents tend to suggest greater innate or genetic causes of their children's violence compared to institutional caregivers; conversely, professional caregivers tend to place more importance on parenting and family dysfunction in causing aggression and violence in young people (ibid.).

The epidemiology of adolescents that are known to have been sexually abusive has identified several risk factors; however, it should be emphasised that much is unknown about young people who abuse other young people. Around one in four adolescents who have been charged with a sexual offence have a 'schedule one' serious sex offender in their family, three out of four had experienced their parents' marital breakdown or divorce, half had been sexually abused before the age of 7 and more than half experienced physical, emotional and/or verbal abuse (Vizard et al. 2007). Within this group, there are high rates of being on the child protection register and having been removed from the family home, with high rates of change of placement, and around two-thirds had histories of being physically or verbally aggressive, or bullying. Clearly, bullying and divorce are far more common than being sexually abusive and are not in themselves risk factors for sexual abuse. However, the over-representation of abusers in comparatively infrequent sub-populations, such as a large number of placements in local authority care, and the combination of many of these risk factors may be indicative of additional need to support young people through their sexual-social development.

The Home Office and Department of Health commissioned a rapid evidence assessment (Itzin et al. 2007) of the literature on the harm to adults relating to exposure to extreme pornographic material (EPM) which included depictions of rape. Based on a modified systematic review methodology it found consistent evidence from experimental studies of aggression after exposure to EPM, the acceptance of rape myths and self-reported likelihood to rape. In particular it focused on the effects of EPM depicting women's sexual arousal and display of pleasure during rape, and the desensitisation, habituation and satiation effects of non-extreme pornographic material on the consumption of EPM. These findings were supported by research with sex offenders. In the UK at least a third of cautioned or convicted sex offenders are adolescents. Case study BP illustrates the impact of pornography effects on an adolescent male who became an adult rapist.

Case study BP: On the aetiology of adult sex offending in adolescence

BP had a conventional childhood until, aged 13, he saw a commercial film in which the beautiful wife of a young professional is brutally abused and raped, and it was difficult for the viewer to determine if the woman was actually resisting and fighting her assaulters or whether she was possibly enjoying the abuse. BP found the actress portraying the woman very sexually attractive and during the rape scenes he produced a full erection. Whenever he thought about the woman he remembered the look on her face as she was being raped, but he could not remember if it was one of pain or pleasure. He fantasised that she could not resist him, that he could force himself upon her and although she might resist, ultimately she gave in to him. He began to develop strong sexual arousal and attraction to forceful sex with adult females and began to masturbate to these fantasies.

At age 14 he began to date females of his own age and although he was strongly attracted to them, he wanted them to be as sexually inviting as the woman in his fantasies, and was surprised when he was repeatedly rebuffed. He returned to masturbating while fantasising about being powerful in sexual relations with adult women. Fantasies about consenting sex were arousing but not as much as those involving rape. After a time he no longer thought about consenting sexual relationships with women.

Before BP performed his first rape, he gained access to pornographic materials in the form of videotapes and magazines which depicted adult women bound, gagged and being sexually humiliated. Similar to his experience with the film at age 13 he could not discriminate whether their expressions were of pain or pleasure. The pornography seemed to reinforce and legitimise rape.

At age 16, BP forcibly raped a 38-year-old woman in the garage of an apartment building. Before the rape he felt he would be able to perform with female peers when he was older. After the rape, he admitted to himself that sexual violence was far more arousing and satisfying. By age 20, BP had raped several women. He had some conventional sexual encounters with women but could only maintain his arousal if he imagined that he was raping them, torturing them or even killing them and he sought out pornography that supported these interests.

(Source: summarised from Laws and Marshall (1990))

Being sexually inappropriate in adolescence is in itself a risk factor for the individual, as well as a risk for those towards whom they may be abusive. Young people who engage in sexually inappropriate behaviour may be at increased risk of exploitation by others. Early victimisation is a particular risk for (re-)victimisation during adolescence. Young people with a history of childhood sexual abuse are at the highest risk for sexual revictimisation in adolescence, and in turn, revictimisation in adolescence increases the risk of revictimisation in adulthood (Classen et al. 2005). Adolescents with sexual abuse histories were up to eleven times more likely to experience rape or a serious sexual assault than those without childhood sexual abuse (Arata 2002). Research carried out in the US identified late adolescence and early adulthood as a particular life phase in which 'risky' sexual behaviours mediate the effects of CSA on later revictimisation (Fargo 2008). Adolescents with sex abuse histories are also more likely to develop sexually inappropriate behaviours during adolescence and to develop sexual offending patterns in adulthood compared to adolescents who have not been abused (Jespersen et al. 2009). However, the development of offending behaviours is not inevitable.

Adolescence is also a risky period for young women to be forced into marriage, around the time of puberty and at an age of 'guaranteed virginity', particularly in cultures that encourage marriage between young women and considerably older men. Factors that may identify a young woman of being at risk of forced marriage and subsequent DV or family violence for resisting the marriage include absence and dropping out from school before the end of compulsory education, and a family history of early marriage, especially older sisters. These issues are explored further in Chapter 7. Cultural factors and patterns of disempowerment of young women may foster vulnerabilities to DV and sexual assault, which in turn emphasises the need for whole community and inter-sectoral action on tackling the exploitation of young people.

Adolescence and a history of sexual abuse in childhood are risk factors for entry into prostitution and sexual exploitation, particularly for those who experience homelessness (which is often brought about by DV), and drug use. Young men are used to groom adolescent girls into prostitution often under the guise of being a boyfriend. This particular pattern of exploitation may be indicated by the boyfriend being older, giving many gifts at the beginning of the relationship, increasing creation of dependency and taking control and isolation from family and friends (Swann 2000). This pattern is indicative of a generally abusive relationship and form of DV, as well as indicating an increased risk for sexual exploitation. Young women who date much older men are also at increased risk of DV, and overall, age-appropriate dating may be a form of prevention from some kinds of exploitation and abuse. Adult offenders also groom adolescent boys, sometimes in similar ways to the grooming of young women, but usually the groomers are older, and the same sex. In general, a history of going missing, running away, homelessness and placement in care are indicative of an increased risk of sexual exploitation and entry into prostitution. Inconsistent or an absence of enrolment in schools and healthcare registration may be indicative of a young person having been trafficked, and as such at high risk of sexual and domestic abuse.

Case study EN: Induction into prostitution

EN began to be groomed by a pimping network after her best friend introduced her when she was just over 11 years old. At 13, she was raped by a gang of men who were part of the pimping network in her town. Mobile phone photographs were taken of these rapes. She then entered prostitution on a regular basis. Shortly after this, she was introduced to drugs; and she began moving drugs for them. She was then passed along to another pimp in the network.

EN went missing from home a number of times. She said, it was fun at first, and when rapes began, she wasn't scared only powerless to resist. As the prostitution developed, there was physical violence. She started to feel frightened when she wanted to testify against the men. She was told that if she spoke out about the pimps, they would kill her – they held a gun to her head, and pulled the trigger; they threatened to kidnap or snatch her from school, kill her family and burn down their house. After this intimidation, she decided to withdraw from prosecution, but she was determined to follow through on her second attempt.

Once the authorities were involved, EN was tested for STDs. She was offered counselling, and a child psychiatrist discussed the possibility following her abuse of borderline personality disorder/schizophrenia as a result of mental trauma. An action plan was set in place to stop sexual abusers from contacting her and she them. Once parents found out, she was constantly monitored: they slept in the same room as her; moved her to a new school; and confiscated the mobile phone which the pimps had given her so they could be in constant contact. Her parents were in regular contact with the police and, as part of the investigation, they collected evidence.

The police,[1] however, lost evidence needed for the court trial. Despite the fact criminal pimping networks are well established and operate in towns in the north of England, they warned EN could be prosecuted for wasting police time; and advised the parents not to contact their MP or newspapers. They said that there was no chance of convicting the men because although they were adult they were 'too young'. Social services remained inactive in the case. EN's school blamed the girl for what had happened to her. And various individual, and multi-agency meetings concluded that it was the parents', not their, responsibility to prevent EN from meeting the pimp network. Furthermore, there was no intervention from their MP.

Since then, a voluntary agency for girls referred EN to social services child protection; and to CROP[2] (when she was 15 years old, nearly four years after the abuse began). They engaged a solicitor who is currently establishing a legal case on the grounds of police negligence. CROP have offered advice and encouragement to her parents and suggested EN write about her experiences.

EN's parents have kept her from re-entering prostitution so far – but, frustrated with the barriers to help, they moved abroad for a couple of years when EN was 16. She has returned to education, but there are still fears for her safety because she is now meeting up with the brother of one of the pimps with whom she was previously involved. This case study illustrates a girl at a later stage of involvement with pimps and a later stage of CROP involvement. CROP's experience is that positive outcomes are much easier to secure at the early stages of pimp involvement, and their assessment is that EN is still very vulnerable to further sexual abuse.

Notes
[1] Police responses vary and new initiatives, such as the Engage multi-agency project in Blackburn, illustrate improved practice.
[2] CROP was founded in 1996 by Irene Ivison whose daughter was coerced into sexual exploitation by a pimp and then murdered by a man paying for sex. From that experience, and that of many other parents, CROP has developed into a national charity with two interrelated objectives. It uniquely supports parents of sexually exploited children and seeks to ensure that their contribution to safeguarding children is included in policy and practice. It also highlights pimping by individual men and criminal networks as those responsible for the commercially driven violent exploitation of children and their families (see www.cropuk.org.uk).
(Case study provided by CROP – printed with permission, EN has now written a book about her experiences (Jackson 2010))

Victims' expectations of health and social sectors

Adolescent victims of abuse and violence need the services they use to be flexible and accessible. They expect, and need, service providers to act honestly, confidentially, respectfully and without judgement, especially as shame and manipulation are important aspects of victimisation. Service providers need to understand about duress and grooming and not blame the victims, or look for complicity in their abuse. The VVAPP Delphi consultation emphasised that young people need flexible and age-appropriate services and materials. 'Flexibility' includes longer opening hours and contact times, as well as drop-in services and administrative systems that do not penalise clients for lateness or missing appointments. This is particularly acute with young people who are homeless, who face multiple vulnerabilities, living with physical, environmental, economic, social and sexual risks. The associations between abuse and poor education attainment have implications for the expected literacy capacity of adolescent clients. Young people who have been victimised are rarely financially independent and costs, both direct and indirect, of attending services should be minimised as much as possible. Confidentiality is essential; however, as offenders who abuse young people often have multiple victims, reporting of abuse may need to be negotiated. As far as possible, abused or victimised young people should be in control of their contact with services, making decisions commensurate with their maturation.

Victims who also display sexually inappropriate behaviours have complex needs to be addressed by the services they access or are referred to, including behavioural issues, psychological symptoms, educational and developmental needs, which are often accompanied by family problems, housing insecurity and other forms of social marginalisation. Often those who display sexually abusive conduct have a history of being abused themselves, and need to have this victimisation recognised and addressed within treatment programmes and efforts to rehabilitate early offenders (Print and Morrison 2000). It is important therefore for services to comprehensively assess new clients, to understand their needs and to develop interventions and support services that respond to those needs.

Effective interventions for victims

One of the limitations of interventions for adolescent victims of abuse and violence is the need for young people to disclose their experiences in order to be matched and admitted to services or programmes, and research suggests that disclosure rates are very low. Additionally, disclosure of abuse experiences is often not made to adults or professionals who can facilitate access to services, but instead is made to friends and peers. A sense of control over disclosure, anticipating that they will be believed and that responses to disclosure will offer choices and effectual support, all contribute to encouraging timely disclosure to appropriate adults (Ungar et al. 2009). Disclosure is particularly unlikely in some of the most at-risk youth, including unaccompanied asylum-seekers and young women from cultures which encourage passivity and silence on 'shameful' experiences (Lay and Papadopoulos 2009).

Young people may be both primary and secondary victims of domestic violence, and may not need their own interventions beyond that which their parents require. While there was general agreement in the VVAPP Delphi consultation that materials and interventions need to be 'age appropriate', there was also caution that chronological age may not be the best indicator of development, capacity or readiness to engage with services. Assessment is therefore important in establishing what the young person needs, can cope with and wants from therapeutic interventions. Young people may benefit from group work and peer support, as well as CBT-type approaches modified to be developmentally appropriate.

Young people who experience sexual abuse or violence need to be assured that they are neither responsible nor to blame for their victimisation. They need interventions and therapies that make them feel safe and believed. As with young people experiencing domestic violence, age-appropriate interventions are important, as well as assessment for their immediate and long-term needs and capacity for therapeutic work. Dissociative disorders need to be considered, and a range of symptoms may be indicative of victimisation, including self-harming or risk-taking behaviours, which also need to be managed within interventions. Re-telling what happened at the point of abuse is not required, and going over details of abuse may be re-traumatising for young people. Instead, adolescent clients should feel in control of the pace, direction and depth of discussion in interventions.

Effective interventions for perpetrators

Two meta-analysis studies of treatment interventions for sex offenders have indicated that interventions with adolescents demonstrate small but positive effects on recidivism, and are more effective than for adults (Losel and Schmucker 2005; Reitzel and Carbonell 2006). Relapse prevention generally has better outcomes for younger offenders (Dowden et al. 2003), and CBT-type interventions that address thought distortion have been identified as producing good treatment outcomes (Walker et al. 2005). Findings from studies of violent adolescents such as Lodewijks and colleagues (2010) indicate that protective factors (such as strong social support, strong attachments and bonds) might mitigate the effects of risk factors in high-risk adolescents, indicating that both risk and protective factors should be targeted in intervention programmes.

A review of current research into the treatment needs and outcomes of young people who sexually abuse others emphasises that this is not a homogenous group (Whittle et al. 2006). Different typologies have been proposed on the basis of victim-choice, offending behaviours, presence of developmental impairment or learning disability, intelligence and educational attainment, and 'personality' traits such as aggression, impulsivity, emotional control and anxiety. With general acknowledgement that not all young people who display sexually inappropriate behaviours go on to be sex offenders, there have also been efforts to identify risk factors for those who are early career offenders, such as persistent and versatile delinquency, histories of conduct disorders and hostility, compared to those whose inappropriate sexual behaviour is resolved by the end of adolescence (Butler and Seto 2002). However, this distinction is complicated by the generally low reporting of abuse carried out by young people and indications that there are broad differences between young people who are 'caught' behaving inappropriately and those who are not, with those in the sexual abuse services during adolescence tending to have higher levels of other psychosocial, developmental, behavioural and conduct problems (Langstrom 2001). Therefore, effective treatments need to be responsive to the holistic needs of the young person at whichever point they enter the support system.

The VVAPP Delphi consultation similarly emphasised the need for interventions to be age-, development- and needs-appropriate, and to be based on an assumption that young people can change their inappropriate behaviours without beginning a deviant or criminal trajectory into adulthood through the development of adaptive and healthy social-sexual conduct and resilience, as well as addressing underlying issues. Residential facilities, which are therapeutic and not punitive, are often useful to provide intense and well-maintained interventions, and to break cycles of behaviour tied to family problems. Alongside this, the experts made clear that the label of sex offenders for young people who display sexually inappropriate behaviours is generally unwarranted and unhelpful. Construing young people, and especially children, as embryonic sex offenders was emphatically rejected.

By comparison, the VVAPP Delphi experts' approaches to interventions for young people who perpetrate DV were somewhat harder, with a greater use of and emphasis on the need for zero-tolerance approaches in treatment and interventions. There were some similarities between the two groups, sexual and domestic, including the need for interventions to be needs-led and tailored to the maturation, learning styles and capabilities of the young client and with the principles of child protection made paramount. Additional parallels between sexual and domestic abusers include: young people who perpetrate domestic violence often have been victims of violence themselves; early intervention is advocated for best treatment outcomes; there is an assumption that young people can change with the right support and resources, and that residential settings may be required for high-risk youth. While anger has been identified as a trigger factor in the perpetration of violence by young people, approaches and interventions that focus purely on anger management were not endorsed by the VVAPP Delphi consultation.

Conclusions

Adolescence is a period of massive change, biological, social, developmental and psychological. The ability for young people to change, both as victims and abusers, is emphasised throughout the research base, and there is an assumption of the potential for resilience, healing and healthy survival of abuse and violence. The need for age- and developmentally appropriate support cannot be underestimated, alongside the need to articulate to young people that the violence and abuses they experience do not define them, and that things that have been perpetrated against them are not their fault or responsibility. Empowerment, safety, belief and respect for the individual are essential for young people to heal and change positively and to resist revictimisation.

5 Violence and abuse across the life-course
Adults

Overview

Adulthood, following adolescence, is the longest phase of the life-course, and represents a period of ongoing development and opportunities for both harm and healing. In adulthood, there is great diversity of pathways into and away from victimisation, revictimisation and sequelae of earlier victimisation, as well as perpetrator trajectories, offending and recidivism. As adults also carry the responsibility for the children in their care, parents are implicated in the response to and prevention of childhood family mal-treatment even when they are not directly abused or abusive. In the later stages of adulthood, parents may become dependent on their children, and the relationships of responsibility shift. Finally, societal level responses to and influences on violence and abuse are generally shaped and reproduced by the adult population, and adults who are neither perpetrators nor victims remain implicated in the shared responsibility for positive values and attitudes towards healthy, safe and respectful interpersonal relationships.

Nature, extent and health effects of domestic and sexual violence and abuse in adulthood

Incidence figures, estimating how often domestic violence occurs and to how many people, are likely to be systematic underestimations. Prevalence surveys across Europe have problems of definition and measurement, and willingness to respond to such surveys, so that data sources that seek to represent IPV are methodologically prone to underestimate the prevalence (Hagemann-White 2001). Most domestic incidents occur away from public view and many adult victims are skilled at hiding the 'evidence' of domestic and intimate partner violence (DV and IPV) as part of managing and containing the abuse. Adults have a range of reasons why they do not report DV and IPV, including shame, fear, confusion, possible stigma and the presence of threats or perceived potential negative consequences of disclosing abuses. These may be consequences for the individual but also for the family unit, and particularly threatening is the perceived likelihood that children will be 'taken away' if DV is revealed. Incidence figures for male victims of DV are particularly difficult to estimate as the phenomenon is broadly under-recognised, and shame and stigma are compounded by disbelief and denial. With regard to sexual assault of males, a nationally representative survey in the US indicated that around 12 per cent of male sexual assault victims report the crime to the police (Light and Monk-Turner 2009).

In the UK, IPV is associated with one quarter of violent crime and an average of two deaths a week. For those aged 18 to 59, around one in four women and one in eight men reported experiencing partner abuse in 2008–09 (HO 2009c). Pregnancy is a particularly risky time, for the initiation and escalation of IPV, and IPV is the leading cause of maternal mortality in the UK, USA and Australia (O'Reilly 2007; Shadigian and Bauer 2005), and as such is preventable. DV and IPV occur in all social strata, but there is some evidence of population disparities, across socio-economic and ethnic groups, and in particular a higher prevalence for learning-disabled people (Field and Caetano 2004; Horner-Johnson and Drum 2006), see also the discussions in Chapters 6, 7 and 8. There is also evidence to indicate that while DV and IPV occur across all socio-economic groups, the inter-sectoral experience of domestic violence as well as poverty, sexism, racism and associated cultural violence compounds the effects of IPV and sustains violence and abuse for marginalised women (Bryant-Davis et al. 2009). For elder abuse and neglect, Cooper and colleagues (2008) carried out a systematic review of studies published up to October 2006. For general population studies, 6 per cent of older people reported significant abuse in the last month and 5.6 per cent of couples reported physical violence in their relationship in the past year. For vulnerable elders (dependent on a carer, disabled), rates were much higher, with nearly 25 per cent reporting significant abuse.

Perpetrators of DV are overwhelmingly male, and in surveys around one in five men admit to using violence, threat, intimidation or similar in their relationships (Mooney 1994, 2000). Broadly, perpetrators of DV are 'normal' men who normally 'get away with it'. However, women also perpetrate IPV, usually less frequently and with less sexual or physical violence compared to male offenders (Reid et al. 2008).

Sexual assault and rape in adulthood is slightly less common than DV for women, with around one in five women aged 18 to 59 reporting this in 2008–09, for men of comparable age the comparable figure is around 1 in 35 (HO 2009c). Non-heterosexual men and women are more likely to experience sexual assault and rape during adulthood, with some evidence suggesting that the risk of sexual assault is doubled for non-heterosexual women and increased by around five times for non-heterosexual men (Todahl et al. 2009). There is an association between IPV and sexual assault, with most offenders being known to the victims, and current and previous partners being particularly over-represented (Finney 2006). While some sexual assaults are precipitated by sexual deviancy and forms of chronic antisocial and hostile behaviours, others are 'regular' men, married with children. Being able to manipulate victims and successfully dominate social situations are important skills in resisting reporting or prosecution.

About 1 per cent of recorded crime in the UK is a sex offence and the majority of known rapes are perpetrated by men. Sexual assault is similarly underreported compared to DV, and grossly under-prosecuted. It is estimated that for each conviction of a sexual offence against children, a perpetrator will have five or more additional offences for which they do not have a conviction (Adi et al. 2002). For information about prevalence of abuse in childhood, please refer to Chapter 2.

Effects of domestic and sexual violence and abuse

The physical and mental health effects of DV and sexual assault can be as varied and broad as definitions of health. Experiencing DV is associated with depression, anxiety, panic attacks, post-traumatic stress disorder (PTSD), as well as chronic pain and function inhibition from injuries (Anderson and Aviles 2006; Bonomi et al. 2006; Whitaker et al. 2006). DV also disrupts employment, education and economic stability, which are determinants of health. Many aspects of feto-maternal mortality and morbidity are associated with DV, including low birth weight, and complications during pregnancy and birth (Boy and Salihu 2004; Leeners et al. 2006; Murphy et al. 2001). Sexual assault is associated with depression, anxiety, panic attacks, PTSD, sexual dysfunction, sleep disorders, irritable bowel syndrome (IBS), and poor sexual health including higher rates of sexually transmitted infections, unwanted pregnancies, repeat abortions and gynaecological problems (Payne 2004; Sarkar and Sarkar 2005; Zimmerman et al. 2006).

For adults who experienced sexual abuse in childhood (CSA), there is an association between CSA and a range of long-term mental health outcomes including dysphoria, depression, low self-esteem, dissociation, sleep disorders, PTSD, suicide ideation and parasuicide, somatisation or bodily distress brought about by psychological distress, avoidance responses including alcohol and substance misuse, and tension reduction behaviours including compulsions and self-harm (Briere and Jordan 2009; MacDonald et al. 2006; Paolucci et al. 2001). A review of studies that considered the association between CSA and psychosis in adulthood concluded that a significant dose-response effect between incidence of CSA trauma and experience of psychosis in adulthood indicates a causal relationship between early childhood sexual trauma and severe mental health outcomes in adulthood (Larkin and Read 2008). Two studies have reported that between 50 per cent and 60 per cent of inpatients and 40 per cent and 60 per cent of outpatients in mental health services have been physically and/or sexually abused as children (Jacobson 1989, Jacobson and Richardson 1987).

Exposure to parental DV in childhood 'potentially leads to poor physical health indirectly through a series of interrelated intermediaries that function along a causal pathway' (Bair-Merritt et al. 2006: 285) as well as associations with poorer mental health outcomes in adulthood. Common across victim groups, victimisation is associated with poor mental health, poor self image and difficulties in building trust (MacDonald et al. 2006). There are also health impacts for non-abusing parents, including the effects of disclosure of abuse on their well-being and parenting, which may occur when the abused child discloses in childhood or later, in adulthood.

Finally, without detracting from the inherent choice and behavioural-decisional basis of offending, perpetrators of IPV and sexual assault also often have unmet health needs, particularly mental health needs including impulse control, and social health needs underlying offending behaviours. There is also an association between engaging in sexually coercive behaviour and risky sexual practices, for example absence of condoms, which in turn are associated with higher rates of sexually transmitted infections, sexual dysfunction, as well as penile and other injuries acquired from resistant and defensive actions by their victims.

Behavioural and self-harming impacts

People who experience DV and sexual assault in adulthood can engage in a range of negative or self-harming behaviours, from rational coping strategies that enable survival of traumatic events but that can have negative effects on other aspects of health, through to intentionally self-destructive behaviours. Experiences of DV and sexual assault are associated with substance abuse and use of drugs and alcohol, and an increase of suicide ideation (Anderson and Aviles 2006). For adults who experienced CSA or were exposed to IPV in childhood, there are associations with suicidal and self-destructive behaviours in adulthood, including alcohol and drug misuse, risk-taking and particularly risky sexual behaviours and unintended pregnancy (Bair-Merritt et al. 2006; Eckhardt et al. 2006). In particular, revictimisation, that is experiencing abuse in childhood and again as an adult, is associated with an increased likelihood of risky sexual behaviours, including sex trading, lack of condom negotiation and multiple partners (Classen et al. 2005). A meta-analysis has suggested that there is a small but positive relationship between experiencing sexual abuse as a child and HIV risk behaviours in later life, including unprotected sex and sex-trading (Arriola et al. 2005). The causal pathways between early sexual and physical abuse and later self-harming behaviours remain unclear, however, and further research is needed to understand what is directly caused by abuse and what co-occurs with the 'event, context and response variables' (Bornstein 2005: 67).

Victims who become abusers and intergenerational effects

Being abused as a child is insufficient to explain or predict perpetration in adulthood. Across multiple generations in the twentieth century, documented patterns of abuse have over-represented girls as victims and men as abusers. If abuse in childhood was an inevitable causal factor of perpetration in adulthood, the proportions would be expected to reverse at some point, which has not occurred. However, the associations between early life victimisation and later perpetration appear to be gendered, with an increased likelihood of boys becoming perpetrators in adulthood than girls, which may suggest that the pathway from victim to perpetrator is mediated by gender roles and social development. Sexuality is also not an appropriate predictor of who becomes an abuser, and although it has been posited, there is no evidence that homosexuality is associated with paedophilia or pederasty. The vast majority of child abusers are heterosexual males, but that is not to say that male heterosexuality should be considered pathological. Instead, it emphasises the need to look beyond simple classifications of gender, sexuality or abuse history to understand the precursors for proclivity to abuse, and in turn the choice to enact offending.

A cycle of family violence is not inevitable. However, there are associations between IPV and forms of family and child physical and sexual abuse which suggest that exposure to perpetration behaviours can be 'passed on'. The likelihood of parental DV is influenced by their early life experiences prior to becoming a parent (Bornstein 2005). Early life exposure to inequitable and abusive relationships can provide persuasive social learning about gender roles and male privilege, learning both how to be manipulative and entitled as well as learning how to be subservient and held responsible for family harmony, broadly along gender lines for boys and girls respectively. A meta-analysis has identified weak to moderate associations between childhood family violence and later IPV experiences, as both perpetrators and victims. This is gendered: boys from IPV backgrounds are more likely to be IPV perpetrators as adults, compared to girls who are more likely to become IPV victims (Stith et al. 2000). Experience of childhood victimisation is a stronger predictor of IPV victimisation in adulthood compared to childhood witnessing of parental DV, which is suggestive of intergenerational effects being amplified by the effects of personal revictimisation.

Protective factors and resilience

Resilience is an important part of surviving abuse and violence, and while there is an unacceptably high homicide and suicide rate associated with victimisation, the prevalence figures indicate that the vast majority of victims do survive their abuse. In addition, not everyone who experiences maltreatment has long-term health effects as a result (Price et al. 2001). Support structures, social, economic and employment security, advocacy and autonomy, access to safety and removal or separation from abuser(s) are important features of resilient contexts in which the impact of abuse may be attenuated. This is not to say that the effects of abuse or the cessation of exposure to violence is the responsibility of the person being abused: abuse is always the responsibility of the perpetrator.

Domestic violence and sexual assault occurs across all social strata, but are more prevalent in societies with greater gender, income and social inequalities; thus resilience can be supported at the societal level as well as the immediate circumstances of the individual (Krahe et al. 2005). Being confident and assertive, with a firm intolerance of violence and low-level emotional or verbal abuse within a social and familial group that shares non-violent norms, may make an individual unappealing to a potentially abusive partner, but essentially the best protection against being abused is not to be in proximity to someone with a propensity to violence and hostility. While adults should not be naive about their peers and potential partners, the burden of prevention of abuse and violence should emphasise social factors, systems and norms that do not facilitate or tolerate abuse, and the importance of individual responsibility for their abusive behaviours and choices.

Victim and survivor expectations

> Often people can seem to want answers, to various issues (for example forgiveness (is it necessary? How do you do it?)) which have no one correct answer and are different for everyone. As a survivor I have found different things helpful at different stages of my healing. In the beginning it was more important that the person who was my support had personal experience of these issues, for me to relate to them and for me to feel they could relate to me and my story. In later years this has mattered less. More important is that I feel that I am accompanied on my journey, in that someone I can tell where I am and my experience, and that can be heard and held.
>
> (Delphi expert)

The Delphi component of the VVAPP identified positive features of health and social care sectors that victims expect to be provided and that make support more accessible. There was broad consensus on the importance of respect for the client, expressed as empathy, regard and warmth, as well as maintaining clear boundaries, working at the pace of the client and expressions of congruence between the worker and the client. Services need to be needs-led and victim-centred, and prefaced by honesty about the demands and limitations of service and intervention options, and be generally solution-focused. The client should be in control of their service use choices and the pace of any interventions they engage with; and client autonomy should be paramount. Findings here are very similar to those obtained by Feder and colleagues (2006) in their meta-analysis of qualitative studies where women who had experienced domestic abuse talked about what they wanted in their interactions with healthcare professionals when their abuse was discussed. For adult survivors of childhood sexual abuse similar findings are also reported in two reviews of the literature (Peleikis and Dahl 2005, Price et al. 2001). Case study NCD illustrates the failure of services to respond appropriately to one DV victim over many years during which her abuse was neither acknowledged nor responded to:

Case study NCD: Adult DV victim failed by services over many years

NCD married at a young age, and first experienced emotional abuse from her husband shortly after her marriage began. She became pregnant and her husband pressured her to have an abortion, citing her 'unfitness' to be a mother, against her wishes. She received no form of abortion counselling, and her wishes were not explored by the abortion clinic. After the abortion, the emotional abuse she experienced intensified as her husband started taunting her with being a 'murderess'. Eventually she consults her GP with psychological distress, antidepressants are prescribed, and she continues on these for 12 years.

She decides to stop taking the anti-depressants (the abuse has not got any better), she does this without support or supervision and suffers a breakdown; she is admitted as a psychiatric in-patient. Throughout all of these health service contacts she is never asked about abuse, or about her perspective on her relationship with her husband. She is reluctant to be discharged home, but the ward staff do not explore the reasons for this, instead encouraging her to return to her 'wonderful' husband, who has been visiting the ward with chocolates etc. for the staff.

She returns home. The abuse intensifies over time. She calls police when she is threatened physically, but receives an unhelpful response that they cannot assist unless she has actually been assaulted; she never calls the police again, even after physical assaults begin. She sought help from the GP to assist her husband in changing his behaviour. On disclosing abuse to her GP, she was not asked about her own needs, or offered any information about services available for herself (she did not ask about these, as she did not envisage that there might be any). No services were arranged for her husband, and the abuse escalated further.

She eventually called the Samaritans, and finally received information about Women's Aid and refuges. The Samaritans arranged a room for her in a refuge, and transport to take her there. She had experienced abuse for over 20 years by this point.

(Source: summarised from Taket et al. (2004))

NCD's case was not an isolated example in the sample of 33 women survivors interviewed by Taket and colleagues (2004). Another six women each reported a similarly long list of contacts with the health service where opportunities to ask direct questions about abuse and home circumstances existed and the circumstances of the consultation indicated that such an enquiry would have been highly relevant. These opportunities were not taken. In some instances women made explicit disclosures, as NCD eventually did to her GP, but this was not followed up with information about relevant services. Cases like this indicate the enormous potential for enabling women to access services at an earlier point in their experience of abuse. Given the prevalence of domestic abuse, such cases also suggest the potential for substantial savings in health service costs. For example, in NCD's case, if she had been able to access appropriate services at an earlier point, potential savings may have included the costs of an extensive length of time on antidepressants, and of her period as a psychiatric inpatient. In contrast, CA's case study was unique among the sample of survivors interviewed (in terms of the comprehensive and coordinated service response achieved), and serves to demonstrate what can be achieved with such a swift and coordinated service response, the important contribution of the voluntary sector, and in particular the benefits of partnership working of statutory and voluntary sector organisations.

Case study CA: A rapid and coordinated response to an adult DV victim and her children

As a child, CA had experienced physical abuse from her father and witnessed her mother's abuse. She married relatively young and had two children, her initial married life was characterised by isolation at home. Abuse commenced soon after the relationship started, but CA had no alternative models of healthy relationships to draw on. It was only when she started taking the children to school and making friends that she realised that 'something was wrong', and that she should not have to tolerate the abuse.

After one episode of physical abuse CA presented at her GP practice with injuries and was given information about a specialist outreach service (run by Women's Aid) available in the practice. An appointment was arranged for the following day. The outreach worker discussed the options available with CA and a few days later CA chose to move into a refuge with her children. While at the refuge she accessed counselling for herself and for the children.

She was given help applying for housing, and relatively quickly was offered a suitable property by the council. She left the refuge after three months for her new home. At time of interview, three months later, she reported positive impacts from services received for both herself and her children.

(Source: summarised from Taket et al. (2004))

Additionally, survivors of DV often want to be kept informed about the progress of their abusers through the judicial system, for example when he will be released from prison or from the police station, and to be given support to meet their children's health and social care needs (DH 2005b). Expecting abused women to take responsibility for ending the violence they experience is unhelpful when the social setting and systems reinforce abuse, including inadequate legal protections, insufficient access to alternative housing and financial support for leaving an abuser, and professionals appearing to minimise abuse or treat calls for help as 'just a domestic' (Bostock et al. 2009). Women who have experienced DV may also benefit from advocacy interventions that are located in healthcare settings, which work towards addressing physical health needs as well as providing safety planning, assistance accessing resources for housing, justice and welfare, and counselling (Hathaway et al. 2008). Domestic violence advocates, when situated with access to a range of economic, housing and safety resources, may be particularly important in meeting the needs of low socio-economic groups and women living in both poverty and domestically abusive settings (Goodman et al. 2009).

Trauma approaches emphasise what has happened *to* an individual rather than emphasising what is wrong *in* them, shifting the locus of the problem from the internal to the external. When delivered in a respectful and client-centred approach, trauma approaches have been identified as particularly helpful for women who have been abused and whose subsequent trauma symptoms have brought them into contact with community mental health services (Harper et al. 2008). In mainstream services, providers need to be aware that adult men and women who have experienced CSA may need increased care in service delivery to achieve positive healthcare experiences, including a higher need for 'informing before performing' and management of triggering situations particularly in intimate examinations (Havig et al. 2008: 27).

Prevention: identifying risk

The health and social care sector are best placed, as the first and frequent point of contact, for identifying people experiencing a range of maltreatment. In primary care, frequent injuries, non-compliance with health advice, signs of anxiety and the unhelpful presence of an interfering partner have all been identified as possible indicators of DV. Additionally, high rates of sexual health issues in women without identity documents may be indicative of being trafficked and a heightened risk of exploitation. Sexual assault co-occurs with DV, with a high proportion of offenders being partners and previous partners, so seeking help for sexual assault may be indicative of further forms of violence as well as a risk factor for revictimisation. General practitioners are often emphasised as best placed for identifying people at risk of being abused, however, other health professionals are also likely to be responding to DV victims. Dental staff and maxillofacial surgeons are likely to have a high proportion of patients who experience DV because of the association between DV and facial injuries, and may need additional training to identify and respond to DV when it is indicated (Coulthard et al. 2004).

The process of identifying people at risk of abuse may be delivered through some well-developed tools of asking about, or screening for, domestic violence and abuse. So far, however, there has been insufficient uptake of these tools to permit evaluation of whether these approaches to enquiring about DV lead to improved health outcomes or reducing risk, and whether screening for DV would be a beneficent process (Nelson et al. 2004; Ramsay et al. 2002; Wathen and MacMillan 2003; Feder et al. 2009). Results of a recent randomised controlled trial of screening in Canada (Macmillan et al. 2009) did examine the question of harm from screening and found that women reported no harm from screening.

It is not only victims that need to be identified as at risk of abuse, but there is also a need to identify perpetrators at risk of abusing, and in particular known offenders who are at risk of reoffending. Going through the judiciary system and being convicted of domestic or sexual assault is insufficient to suggest that the perpetrator has the skills and the preferences to avoid reoffending, and broadly the absence of engagement with a rehabilitation or offence-specific intervention may indicate a continued risk of perpetration. Social deviance, including antisocial conduct, poor impulse control, rule violations and hostility; and sexual deviance, including a preference for sex with children or rape, are indications of a heightened risk of perpetrating violence or abuse. Those most at risk of sexually reoffending are 'not upset or lonely; instead he leads an unstable, antisocial lifestyle and ruminates on sexually deviant themes' (Hanson and Morton-Bourgon 2005: 1158).

Referral and risk management

The identification of risk is insufficient in itself; there need to be pathways to help support safety and change, and the risk, once identified, needs to be managed, contained and ameliorated. Training and awareness of local options is needed for service staff, and the system needs to be collaborative to facilitate progression from identification to referral (Ramsay et al. 2005). The Delphi component of the VVAPP highlighted that victims and those at continuing risk of assault and abuse need access to relevant services and advocacy, and may benefit from referrals from helplines and charities as well as health and social care services. Feder and colleagues' systematic review (2009) includes a review of quantitative studies of advocacy interventions. The review finds a number of studies that show some benefit from advocacy for some outcomes, in terms of reduction of abuse, increases in social support, increases in quality of life and increased use of safety behaviours and accessing community resources. Where a recent sexual assault is disclosed, immediate referral to forensic services is indicated. For perpetrators of violence and abuse, there is a need for voluntary places in interventions not just mandated places, so that perpetrators who want to change are not excluded from rehabilitation and that help is not dependent on conviction.

The VVAPP Delphi consultation also identified important features of risk management strategies, with a high degree of consensus on the need for the establishment of safety as the first priority. Confidentiality is important but needs to be balanced with prioritising child protection strategies, which may need to supersede the confidentiality of the adult individual. For perpetrators, risk management similarly entails a priority of safety and child protection, and good interventions were identified as being risk-led, with risk and safety superseding client-centred, needs-led approaches, which may not be risk-appropriate, particularly at the point of identification and referral.

Three individual circumstances may be considered as identifying being at risk of abuse or violence: being learning disabled, having a history of childhood abuse and having a recent history of assault or abuse. Learning-disabled people may be at an increased risk of assault and abuse, and this risk can be managed through the regulation of workers and carers (for example, accreditation and background checks) as well as interventions aimed at empowering the individual. Protection skills are most effective when they are developed along three dimensions – knowledge including sex education and the right to say 'no', role play to rehearse identifying threatening situations and resistance strategies, and feedback or assessment of people's responses to threats. Empowering interventions that teach and encourage assertiveness and the use of 'stop' and 'no' to assert a client's autonomy may, in the short term, be in conflict with care environments that expect and reward compliance. Staff training and needs assessment of the individual client are important to support appropriate protection skill development programmes and enable authentic strategies for the individual (Bruder and Stenfert Kroese 2005).

Two meta-analyses have considered the effects of early victimisation on the likelihood of later revictimisation (Classen et al. 2005; Roodman and Clum 2001). The experience of childhood sexual abuse increases the chances of adult revictimisation, with up to two-thirds of CSA victims experiencing sexual assault in adulthood. For women, CSA doubles the likelihood of sexual revictimisation, and for men there is evidence that the effect is even stronger, being around five times more likely to be revictimised. There is some indication that severity of first abuse, use of force at first abuse and length of first abuse, as well as the relationship with the first abuser may be associated with later patterns of victimisation. This may be cumulative, so that people with more victimisation events and more abusers are increasingly at risk of further revictimisation. Multiple revictimisation is associated with worse mental outcomes, including higher levels of PTSD and increased likelihood of dissociation; in turn, severe mental health problems are associated with increased risk of revictimisation. Revictimisation with multiple abusers is associated with delayed disclosure, which in turn is associated with longer periods of being at risk and delays in the provision of safety and recovery. For women who have experienced CSA and prostitution in adulthood, there is an increased risk of poor mental health outcomes and PTSD symptoms (Choi et al. 2009). Case study AE illustrates the patterns and characteristics found in the literature.

Case study AE: Incest, paedophilia, prostitution, pornography: organised familial, extrafamilial and intergenerational abuse

AE described herself as born illegitimate and premature, probably the child of incest between her mother and her mother's father, her grandfather. Her mother abused her physically and emotionally, and her mother and her grandmother would actually send her to be abused by her grandfather. She said her stepfather did not abuse her: that he was fabulous, and still was. But he worked all hours and didn't know what was going on. She was abused by her mother's younger brothers, her uncles, when they were babysitting and they told her they'd been taught by their father, her grandfather. Her uncles would make her look at pornographic literature and then take photographs of her doing it naked. They used to sell her to their friends and charge them to have sex with her. This was from the age of four to eleven.

In her early childhood, in addition to the incest at home, she'd be taken to places for group sex, group pornography, group prostitution. She described a network of people whose paths crossed for these purposes. No one ever told her not to say anything, not ever, but she said she knew she shouldn't.

When her family moved to live next door to her grandparents and aunts and uncles, the sexual abuse accelerated, and the pornography properly started with a friend of her grandfather who photographed children. There were groups of other children and adults and group sex and she would be made to be a perpetrator and sexually abuse younger children through oral sex or penetrating their vagina or rectum. There were babies involved too. In the pornography there was also violence, tying up, and restraint. There was also recording. Afterwards the children would be given sweets.

Her fear was always that the photographs of her would turn up. When she was in her twenties, her uncle showed her some he still had, of her at age nine. She described her response as total horror – at how small she was, her eyes were dead but she was smiling. They'd told her to smile. She'd learned from an early age that total obedience was required. When they finished with her, she used to say thank you. The reward was being a good girl. That was the only affection she ever got and she'd do anything for it. She let herself be abused by a variety of men for the reward of being called a good girl, sexual activities had become the norm.

She didn't even know it was wrong until, training as a nurse, she went to a lecture on sexually transmitted diseases and learned that incest was illegal. From that moment, it just felt devastating. Everything she'd done and felt she'd had to do she discovered that she didn't have to do, that most people don't have to do it, but she had. She was then to discover the enormity of the damage done to her in terms of self-harm (cutting, self-mutilation, eating disorders), mental illness requiring 25 years of psychotherapy and ten years of admissions for psychiatric inpatient treatment, attempted suicide. She said it was very hard for her children.

She said in spite of what they'd done to her, she doesn't hate them, she loved them because they were her family When a friend told her recently that she would have rescued her and adopted her if she had found her as a child, she said she wouldn't have wanted rescuing, She wanted her own family and her biggest terror was that somebody would take her away and put her with strangers. She said the chances of her telling anyone as a child would have been remote because she would only have told someone if she was absolutely sure they were going to be sympathetic to all of the family and not just her. She said she would rather have had the abuse than not have her family.

(Source: summarised from chapter 7 in Itzin (2000))

Although there are clear associations between early victimisation in childhood and revictimisation in adulthood, it is unclear whether childhood sexual abuse or childhood physical abuse are stronger predictors of revictimisation or what their relative roles may be in increasing the risk of victimisation in adulthood. There is some emerging evidence of a recency effect, indicating a possible risky period after victimisation that attenuates over time. While this is still tentatively theorised at the moment, it highlights the need for timely responses to victims, both for their recovery and healing but also for protecting against further experiences of abuse.

Effective interventions for perpetrators

From a study of interventions for men who perpetrated domestic abuse (Buchbinder and Eisikovits 2008: 619), this is how a man who had undergone approximately ten months of therapy and was about to be released from jail described the changes that took place during his treatment process:

INTERVIEWEE: … I felt more relaxed. I spoke more, hard stuff that touched also my most intimate, personal life … I actually mean the most negative things in my inner self, a considerable part of me that took over my entire self. What was I like, after all? I was into delinquency, I was into crime, I was into murky business, I was into violence against my family, violence against both the wife and outsiders because I was living within rigid frames, a mentality of principles and honor ... Here, I actually connected with my feelings. I hadn't known what feeling was. I can tell you, even more deeply – it was here that I felt the joy of living. Even though this is a prison, a closed framework, this is where I started feeling; I started feeling the joy of life, the openness ... Actually, it allowed me to process who I would like to be. Do I really want to continue like this because it is comfortable for me or could I also be different and determine my character by myself?

INTERVIEWER: What is your answer to yourself?

INTERVIEWEE: Today I tell myself one thing: although I [silence] – I am not going to win this woman back. But I won more than that – myself. I was privileged to be able to gain myself.

In a needs-led and victim-centred model, risk management focuses on the protection and resilience of the individual victim. However, this needs to be balanced by the onus of responsibility for abuse being focused on the perpetrator, and the safety-needs of the community in which he lives and offends. A meta-analysis of interventions for adult sex offenders has indicated that psychological treatment produces a small but positive effect, both for sexual and general recidivism (Hanson et al. 2002). Features of successful interventions with adult sex offenders, that is those that reduce the risk of reoffending, include identifying high-risk situations and role play (Dowden et al. 2003), which is interestingly similar to features of good practice in interventions that seek to reduce risk by enabling learning-disabled people to protect themselves against abuse and victimisation. There is a need for interventions with sex offenders to identify and seek to replace maladaptive conduct, more rigorously reducing offending than simply seeking to provide offenders with ways of suppressing offending behaviours (Simons et al. 2008). In evaluations of the Clearwater Program (a high-intensity sex offender treatment programme in a Canadian federal maximum security correctional treatment facility), three factors have been identified in the successful reduction of recidivism through high-intensity inpatient intervention: the matching of intensity of intervention to the assessed risk of reoffending; needs-specific treatment priorities; and responsive tailoring of the intervention to their capacity and motivations for engaging with the intervention (Olver et al. 2009). This programme has included medium- to high-risk offenders, and has approximately halved the long-term recidivism rate compared to a control group over a 20-year period as measured by reconviction for a sexual offence (ibid). A meta-analysis (Dowden et al. 2003) of relapse prevention programmes for offenders (a variety of offender types were included within the analysis, not solely perpetrators of sexual or domestic violence) found moderate mean reductions in recidivism and that particular elements of the relapse prevention model yielded stronger effects than others. In particular the effects of training significant others and identifying the offence chain were stronger than those of booster/aftercare sessions and developing coping skills.

There is no clear evidence that learning-disabled people are over-represented in sex offender figures; however, there is some indication that learning-disabled offenders have particular needs for effective treatment, including sex education and social competencies (Lindsay 2002). There is a tendency for mainstream interventions primarily aimed at male offenders to be modified for other groups, such as women or learning-disabled people. Some features of mainstream interventions, and in particular CBT-type treatment, may be problematic for learning-disabled people, although there is also some evidence that aspects of CBT such as the use of labelling of behaviours rather than abstract reasoning or reflection, may be helpful (Wilcox 2004). The Adapted Sex Offender Treatment Programme for people with low IQ or learning disability (a treatment programme for people with low IQ or learning disability that combines CBT, impulse control and sex education, which has been run in five English prisons) combines CBT, impulse control and sex education, and there is emerging evidence that the combination of CBT with social skills training is most appropriate for low-risk learning-disabled sex offenders (Barron et al. 2002). There is also some indication that longer treatment is associated with better outcomes for learning-disabled adult sex offenders (Courtney and Rose 2004).

At the other end of a spectrum of offending, high-risk sex offenders and in particular those who do not respond to psychosocial interventions have been treated with castration treatments. A meta-analysis indicates that castration treatments, surgical or medicated, have better treatment effects and lower recidivism than psychosocial treatments (Losel and Schmucker 2005). However, this is at least partly explained by differences in offenders that undergo different kinds of treatments, and the comparative rarity of castration interventions. Medical castration may also increase the risk of recidivism at the point of drop-out or discontinuation of treatment, which may be indicative of the client being at continued underlying risk of offending that is not necessarily minimised but rather restrained by treatment. There is some emerging evidence that selective serotonin reuptake inhibitors (SSRIs) may be useful in the treatment of sex offenders, which lower libido without being a form of castration, as well as being mood-altering (Adi et al. 2002), however, this treatment has not been adequately demonstrated as effective for particularly high-risk offenders. A systematic review of the effects of Luteinising Hormone Releasing Hormone (LHRH) agonists as a method of chemical castration indicated fewer side effects compared to earlier types of drugs, and general efficacy of reducing recidivism for sex offenders, while under treatment, that exceeded SSRIs and older chemical castration drugs (Briken et al. 2003).

Overall, clients who volunteer for castration treatment have more effective outcomes than those who do not volunteer, but again this may be partly explained by differences between offenders who have the option and those for whom the treatment is mandated, as well as possible skewed patterns in adherence and drop-out (Losel and Schmucker 2005).

Psychosocial interventions for perpetrators of domestic violence, such as those used by the judicial system for the risk-reduction and rehabilitation of convicted DV offenders, have been shown to have a small but positive effect on recidivism (Babcock et al. 2004), although it is important to note that many kinds of DV interventions are outside the scope of published evaluations and are not represented in meta-analysis of treatment effects. Examples of unevaluated DV interventions, such as pastoral interventions carried out by faith leaders, are discussed further in Chapter 9 on abuse by professionals. For men who are legally required to attend an IPV perpetrators intervention there is a reduction of around 5 per cent in recidivism, compared to men with similar convictions that are not compelled to attend an intervention as part of their sentencing (Feder and Wilson 2005). Men who drop out from IPV perpetrators inventions are more likely to reoffend than those who complete the intervention (ibid.) and drop-out from treatment may be a likely marker of recidivism risk (Hanson et al. 2002). It remains unclear what the important features of an effective DV intervention may be, and greater differences in recidivism outcomes can be found in the methodology used to measure recidivism (partner reports or police incident reports) than in the method of intervention, for example cognitive behavioural, couples' therapy or close monitoring (Eckhardt et al. 2006). The lack of significant differences between treatment approaches, for example CBT-type and power and control, Duluth-type models, may be an artefact of the lack of applied differences between the two labels and overlap of theory and treatment practices (Babcock et al. 2004). Qualitative studies with men who have been in IPV interventions suggest that some men learn how to cope with their aggression through the intervention but that this leads to a temporary suppression of violence which is not sustained. Those who revise their self-identity and develop an authentic sense of a non-violent self are more likely to find interventions successful and sustain reductions in violence. However, the process of developing an authentic non-violent self generates a lot of anxiety and reassessment of core self values, which is confronting for men and requires additional care from the intervention to sustain treatment, and replace the violence with something positive, attainable and authentic (Buchbinder and Eisikovits 2008).

Case study PP: DV perpetrator effective intervention

PP grew up with many silences and secrets engineered by adults, with his grandfather maimed in World War I and who, he later found out, eventually committed suicide. His father had been injured and disabled in World War II, an experience simply never spoken of, nor did he speak of the death of his father. PP shared how additionally shocked he was to learn only a few years previous that his mother's current marriage to his father was her second marriage.

Disclosure, then, was something of which he had little experience, and he learned the familial culture of secret-keeping. He also learned to repress his vulnerability and to make such repression as part of his masculinity: he recollected how his father hit him upon being told he was being bullied at school, and how he understood this as a lesson in the importance of not crying. PP attended a therapeutic perpetrator programme, with up to 12 individual sessions followed by 48 group sessions. PP saved his marriage through his participation on the programme, he was excited about his participation.

He discussed the programme almost entirely in the context of how he changed with each recollected moment, and ascribed great importance to how supportive the other men in the group had been, he considered the group's support in working through feelings as the main vehicle for his improvement. PP said how 'incredible' it was to be able to talk about feelings, and how rare it was 'as a man' to talk about feelings, which everyone 'poo-poos'. His wife overheard the phone interview and corrected small details (e.g. age of children, manner of referral); he happily put her on the phone to discuss programme impact on relationships; she said he still has a 'short fuse' and he shouts, but he generally realises what he has done within an hour and apologises. PP, however, did not label his behaviour as abusive, yet admitted in the same language as his wife to 'small problems' they are working on.

(Source: summarised from Garfield (2007), used with permission.)

Effective therapies and interventions for victims

> And sometimes you still get down, but I know when I'm down without a shadow of a doubt, I'm going to come back. I'm happier now. ... In one of my things I wrote at college – ... I [wrote] 'I was somebody's wife, I was somebody's mother and then I was somebody's possession and, *now, I'm me*' [emphasised]. That you should put down because that I feel is relevant.'
>
> ('Jean', Wakefield, domestic abuse survivor who had accessed multiple services including counselling and support groups, talking about her experience of the effects of this service use, research participant interviewed in study reported in Taket et al. 2004)

The VVAPP Delphi consultation identified core principles and features of good practice in effective, appropriate and safe interventions for victims of DV and sexual assault. These include a primacy of safety, and the need to protect the client's privacy and confidentiality. At the start of the therapy or intervention, service providers should hold assumptions of believing the client, assuming that reports of abuse and violence are serious and that clients do not need to describe the details of abusive incidents as a prerequisite for engaging in therapy. Through the course of the therapy/intervention, it is important for the direction and pace of the process to be guided by the client, following an individual course, which is often most helpful to consider as a toolkit approach. The individual therapist should work towards developing a congruent relationship with the client, that is one that shares similar aims, facilitates trust, seeks to empower the client, and is characterised by attentiveness, listening and not blaming the client. A therapeutic intervention should seek to address underlying problems, beyond symptoms; and those symptoms particularly associated with self-destructive behaviours should be respected as coping strategies that need to be replaced rather than simply problems to be erased. Feder and colleagues' systematic review (2009) includes reviews of a number of different types of intervention for women who have experienced partner abuse; the review was confined to quantitative studies only. The strongest evidence was found for individual psychological interventions. For group psychological interventions and support groups, although there was some evidence of positive effects, weakness in study execution mean that evidence of effectiveness is not so strong.

The guidelines commissioned by the VVAPP on *Psychoanalytic Psychotherapy after Child Abuse* (McQueen et al. 2008) covers the effects of childhood abuse and neglect on adult survivors such as insecure and disordered attachments, trauma and dissociation, dissociative disorders, affect regulation and post-traumatic stress disorders. It brings together for the first time the evidence base for the effectiveness of psychoanalytic psychotherapies and their processes and applications, including assessment, patient–therapist interaction and the importance of the therapeutic alliance in the treatment of adults (and children) who have experienced sexual abuse, violence and neglect in childhood.

Many of the Delphi experts offered strong support for the use of integrated or mixed approaches, the view that there is no single approach that is best for everyone, and that different approaches each have their place in a staged process of intervention. Stages were typically conceptualised by the respondents as three phases: (1) establishing safety and stabilising; (2) dealing with traumatic memories and addressing psychological harm; (3) reconnecting and rebuilding a post-abuse life, without, however, implying simple sequential ordering in this process. This process involves drawing flexibly on a range of different approaches according to stage and circumstances/context, based on characteristics of victim/survivor-centredness, and stressing the importance of the quality of the therapeutic relationship, and of non-judgementality. A detailed example of a three-stage approach put forward as applicable to adult victims/survivors of rape and sexual assault *and* domestic violence is summarised in Figure 5.1.

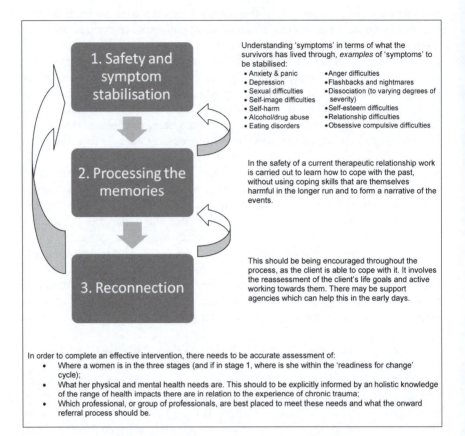

Figure 5.1 illustrates a three-stage approach:

1. Safety and symptom stabilisation

Understanding 'symptoms' in terms of what the survivors has lived through, *examples* of 'symptoms' to be stabilised:
- Anxiety & panic
- Anger difficulties
- Depression
- Flashbacks and nightmares
- Sexual difficulties
- Dissociation (to varying degrees of severity)
- Self-image difficulties
- Self-harm
- Self-esteem difficulties
- Alcohol/drug abuse
- Relationship difficulties
- Eating disorders
- Obsessive compulsive difficulties

2. Processing the memories

In the safety of a current therapeutic relationship work is carried out to learn how to cope with the past, without using coping skills that are themselves harmful in the longer run and to form a narrative of the events.

3. Reconnection

This should be being encouraged throughout the process, as the client is able to cope with it. It involves the reassessment of the client's life goals and active working towards them. There may be support agencies which can help this in the early days.

In order to complete an effective intervention, there needs to be accurate assessment of:
- Where a women is in the three stages (and if in stage 1, where is she within the 'readiness for change' cycle);
- What her physical and mental health needs are. This should to be explicitly informed by an holistic knowledge of the range of health impacts there are in relation to the experience of chronic trauma;
- Which professional, or group of professionals, are best placed to meet these needs and what the onward referral process should be.

Figure 5.1 Outline of a three-stage approach for adult victims/survivors of rape and sexual assault or domestic violence.

For victims of sexual assault, good practice involves meeting the immediate health and trauma needs of clients as well as forensic responsibilities, and longer-term healing and therapeutic needs; in the UK, Sexual Assault Referral Centres (SARCs) were highlighted as examples of good practice in the short-term care of rape and sexual assault victims, with referral points to opt in to further support as necessary. For victims of domestic violence, the Respect framework was highlighted as an example of good practice. For adult survivors of childhood sexual abuse the Survivor's Trust member organisations provide specialist counselling, advocacy and other support services locally, regionally and nationally.

Given the mental health sequelae of abuse and victimisation, good practice in the mental health sector is particularly important, and as an alternative entry point to support and intervention outside of primary health settings, mental health professionals have a particular responsibility and position to align victims with appropriate support for underlying histories of victimisation when presenting symptoms known to be associated with experiencing abuse and violence. Asking patients in mental health settings about experiences of IPV can encourage disclosure (Wathan and MacMillan 2003) and for adults who experienced sexual abuse in childhood, the diagnosis and treatment of dissociative disorders can be an important part of the therapeutic process. Mental health services are also important for the appropriate treatment of perpetrators including screening for mental health issues and readiness for engagement in interventions, and providing treatment for other mental health and addiction needs.

Case study 'Susan': Dissociation and successful therapeutic intervention

Susan was 26 when she was referred by both a counsellor from her GP practice and a locum psychiatrist from the hospital where she had been sectioned.

Although she had lengthy medical files showing urinary infections, stomach complaints, unexplained periods of depression, and two in-patient periods after A levels and then after her degree, she had nevertheless succeeded in becoming a junior school teacher and expressed great satisfaction with her job.

On the morning of Halloween, October 31st, after she had been in post for three years, a child from her class had a mild concussion after falling from a swing in playtime. Even though the child recovered, with mild concussion, and she had not been the teacher on playground duty, she felt profoundly guilty. She could not sleep, found herself crying and became beset with terrible images of children being hurt. Her sympathetic GP provided her with mild sleeping pills and referred her to the practice counsellor.

Susan spoke for the first time of her abusive family. There were also neighbours and cousins who somehow fitted into her narrative through a shared abusive belief system that traumatised the GP counsellor. As punishment for speaking Susan started hearing a voice in her head that told her she was evil and a child-killer. She had to take sick-leave from her job, became increasingly suicidal, and was hospitalised.

Aided by a locum psychiatrist who considered that the injured child had re-activated a dormant dissociative state, she decided to seek a specialist referral aided by her GP counsellor and the psychiatrist. In treatment, Susan slowly realised that she had needed dissociation to survive the cult abuse by family and others in her childhood. It was an alter-personality, Sarah, who had gone to college and undertaken the teaching diploma and a terrified and furious child alter, Mad, who had made the threatening statements. Mad, an 8 year old, had to identify with the abusing cult family in order to survive and had been made to feel he had committed the murder of a child on Halloween. As treatment progressed, Mad changed his name to Max and decided he would be a great protector of children. Susan and Sarah expressed a wish to join together but Max remained separate.

Coming to psychotherapy at such a young age and with abuse having totally stopped at the age of 18, Susan had a good prognosis, and after the first two years of intensive psychotherapy was able to return to her job.

(Source: Case Study provided by Clinic for Dissociative Studies: this has merged two clients' experiences with their permission)

There is a need for a whole system approach to responding to with the range of perpetrators and victims across multiple forms of abuse and violence. The need for a multi-sectoral approach to service delivery, with strong collaboration between different agencies, is clearly illustrated in the case studies throughout this book, and the discussions in Chapters 7 and 8 in particular.

Other services that may be important for responding to, managing and treating abuse and victimisation include: confidential helplines, charities that provide information, advocacy, accommodation and referrals to services, peer-led support groups including internet-based communities, and drug, alcohol and self-harm support services. The wider community is also implicated in tackling the root causes of violence, and a whole system approach needs to be embedded in societal attitude changes. This was emphasised particularly strongly by the Delhi experts:

I do not believe that true prevention is possible in western society as it is currently constructed since it requires a major shift in political and public consciousness, in gender roles and the redistribution of power between men, women and children. Within the current construction of society, a political lead is needed towards ... where every child is wanted and its needs provided for (via social and welfare provision), and towards the creation of a culture where no form of violence, from war to smacking children, is socially and legally sanctioned and tolerated.

(Delphi expert)

The issues of lack of funding, lack of political will, lack of priority and lack of public visibility and the need for societal wide action come through in every single programme area – along with support for a broad public health approach and the need for an integrated high-profile national strategy (with some differences about the extent to which integration is possible/desirable). It was emphasised that policy-makers need to resist the temptation to impose unitary solutions to the huge diversity of different situations and recognise that the keys to successful policies are likely to be sensitivity and flexibility.

A number of responses noted the lack of a joined-up approach at national level, suggesting that this be addressed through a comprehensive national strategy that recognises the need for action in all sectors of society. Particular components that were stressed were:

- Need for widespread change in public attitudes and knowledge about the extent and nature of abuse – keeping an appropriate balance between the coverage of 'stranger danger' and abuse by known and trusted adults, with recognition that men are also victims/survivors of sexual violence and abuse. Alongside this runs the need to 'challenge the silence about sexual abuse'.
- Need for government departments to work with the media to give clear messages that people can recognise and take appropriate action about abusive behaviours.
- Need to challenge the problem that abuse not seen as relevant in NHS settings, e.g. not a 'mental health' issue. This relates to services still being organised around diagnostic categories and medical models of care where links are not made between experience of abuse and presenting distress or 'symptoms'. 'Once a person has a diagnostic label (e.g. ADHD, Personality Disorder, OCD etc.) there is no need to ask any more questions, which inhibits disclosure.' (Taket and Barter-Godfrey 2006: 113)

As well as good practice, the Delphi consultation also identified practices that were not necessarily helpful and had the potential to be harmful or counterproductive. These include approaches that rely exclusively on medication or exclusively on behaviour, and strategies that involve reenactment, visualisation or regression to times of abuse. Generally directive and prescriptive approaches were seen as unhelpful (a conclusion replicated in the professional abuse chapter around pastoral DV counselling), including but not limited to, strategies that demand forgiveness as part of the therapeutic process or that *demand* the use of touch or holding. For offenders, forms of collusion with, or minimisation of perpetration, are constructed as particularly inappropriate.

Areas of mixed views

There were substantial areas of agreement throughout the Delphi consultations; however, there were also some areas in which there was disagreement about what is effective and appropriate. These broadly fell into two areas: dynamics between needs and safety within family units and practice issues for specific client groups.

The role of family therapy and the involvement of perpetrators and victims within the same intervention were particularly contentious. There are problems with the management of safety and risk attributed to the presence of a known perpetrator, particularly prior to the perpetrator having engaged in addressing his own behaviours, and doubts over the likelihood that an intervention can be empowering, safe and truthful for victims when perpetrators are integrated, and thus at least partly in control of a family intervention. However, a family does not become a void in the wake of family violence and new, healthy family dynamics are needed to replace violent and abusive behaviour patterns, and as such, family interventions may have a role in long-term healing and rehabilitation after DV. These issues were particularly acute in whether and where to put children in family interventions (as discussed in Chapter 3). The role of reconciliation within DV interventions was similarly contentious, with tensions between the need to support the survivor/victim in exerting their autonomy and making choices about their relationships, and the service provider's need to protect their client from a known source of harm.

For specific client groups and settings, there was a lack of agreement over the use of treatment aids, ranging from uncertainty about the use of 'survivor literature' for adult victims of childhood sexual abuse, through to the usefulness of psychotropic medication for adult victims of DV, and the use of chemical castration for sex offenders. Across these different positions there was a noticeable emphasis on the importance of treatment choices being responsive to the needs and capacities of the individual client, and an understanding that there is no single blueprint intervention that is effective for all clients. However, in one area the preferences of individual clients may be in conflict with the needs of other service users, and the best placement of male victims of rape and sexual assault, within or separate from women's sexual assault services, was unclear. This uncertainty over the need for gender segregation in services, juxtaposed with a need for equality in access to services has raised debate and problems of application of the Gender Equality Duty and the Single Equality Duty (Equality and Human Rights Commission 2006, 2008), and in particular whether local authority funded organisations providing services to women experiencing domestic violence also have to provide the same services to men.

For perpetrators of DV, there was some disagreement over the use of anger management, and the role of anger/impulse control in the aetiology of DV, compared to, or in conjunction with, issues of power, control and privilege. A variety of different positions emerged on the role of group work for offenders, and the order in which individual and group work should occur.

Conclusions

> I left after 48 years of marriage of which I suffered 33 years of verbal abuse. Women's Aid gave me a new life at 71. [After] about a month of contact with Women's Aid I was in my own flat and at peace for the first time in many years. Three and a half years on, they are still there

when I need them, no praise is high enough for the women who run this service ...

(Questionnaire respondent, Salford, on her experience, quoted from Taket et al. 2004: 51)

There is a strong evidence base that explicates the health outcomes for victims of abuse and violence in adulthood, as well as the amplifying effects of revictimisation. Some of the pathways between instances of abuse and specific sequelae remain unclear, although this is at least partly because of the complexity of the interrelationships between individual and situational factors for both the perpetrator and victim in creating the immediate experience and subsequent effects for the survivor. Similarly, there is a strong evidence base that demonstrates the need for, and successes of, interventions to reduce recidivism; however, the specific causal pathways between offender and cessation of offending remain unclear, and some treatment options remain contentious or unproven. As with previous chapters, there is an emphasis on inter-sectoral action, protection, safety and confidentiality as guiding principles for victim-centred services; and the need for containment of abuse, challenging abuse-facilitating beliefs and addressing social and sexual deviance for perpetrators.

Part III

Addressing inequalities

Specially commissioned chapters within the third part of the book examine key factors that are important in understanding how and why different groups experience heightened risks of violence and abuse, and the factors important in shaping appropriate responses to their needs. These chapters examine: gender and sexuality, race and culture; disability; and abuse by professionals. These chapters explore how some of the general principles discussed earlier can be applied appropriately to the specific needs of the individual, taking into account how these are shaped by the interactions between culture, ethnicity, social position, gender, sexuality, disability and society.

6 Gender and sexuality

Marianne Hester

Introduction: gender, sexuality and inequality

This chapter addresses the gendering of interpersonal violence and abuse; and the implication of sexuality for the experience of interpersonal violence and abuse by heterosexual, lesbian and gay individuals.[1] While the literature on violence and abuse often considers gender and sexuality as separate issues and phenomena, processes of gendering and issues related to sexuality are by no means discrete. Here some of the overlaps, links and implications of difference will also be considered. Understanding how gender and sexuality intersect with regard to how individuals may use, experience and embody violence and abuse enables a comparison of similarities and differences across abusive lesbian, gay male or heterosexual relationships, and to consider possibly different experiences and different needs for these groups of individuals with regard to health and mental health interventions.

Gender and inequality

Gender is a key feature in patterns of interpersonal violence and abuse. Who abuses whom and how is underpinned by gender inequality. Meanings attributed to, and expectations associated with, gender also impact on the ways in which professional approaches to perpetrators, victims or survivors, adults and children are played out. Gender is of crucial importance to understanding the impact of interpersonal violence and abuse on individuals, and understanding what may work in overcoming victimisation. At the same time, sexuality – where individuals identify as heterosexual, or as lesbian or gay – creates different experiences and outcomes (as may age, class, race, disability – see other chapters). In heterosexual contexts, constructions of power and violence are highly gendered, and linked to culturally constructed and idealised forms of masculinity and femininity – what has been termed 'hegemonic masculinity' and 'hegemonic heterosexuality' (Connell 1987). The social construction of masculinity, as embodied in heterosexual men, helps to explain, for instance, domestic violence as the exertion of power and control by men over women in intimate relationships within contexts of gender inequality (Hester 2004).

In same-sex relationships gender is not as prominent in positioning individuals within relationships and in interactions and constructions of power and violence. There is, however, still evidence of gendered norms impacting on experiences and outcomes of violence and abuse for lesbians and gay men (Hester and Donovan 2009). This will be explored alongside the discussion of gender throughout this chapter.

Stark (2007) focuses more specifically on the processes of gender inequality involved in violence and abuse, calling the processes involved in domestic violence, prostitution and other forms of heterosexual violence against women 'coercive control'. Drawing on research into hostages as well as work with women who have experienced abuse from male partners and others, Stark argues that theories highlighting power and control do not go far enough. Instead, he uses the idea of coercive control, as this is where the individual aims specifically (in instances of domestic violence) 'to usurp and master a partner's subjectivity' (ibid.: 205). He concludes 'The result is a condition of unfreedom (what is experienced as *entrapment*) that is "gendered" in its construction, delivery and consequence' (ibid.: 205). The violence used in coercive control:

> ... is designed to punish, hurt or control a victim; its effects are cumulative rather than incident-specific; and it frequently results in severe injury or death. ... the victim's susceptibility to injury is a function of the degree to which her capabilities for defence, resistance, escape or to garner support have been disabled by a combination of exploitation, structural constraints and isolation.
>
> (Stark 2007: 205)

Taking a wider, historical, view, of violence, abuse and gender, Hester (1992) argues that violence and abuse 'work' and impact on individuals to sustain, create and recreate social inequalities. The use as well as threat of violence and abuse has the effect of controlling individuals' lives, and serves, within the context of gender inequality, to construct men as more powerful than women. Thus, violence against women serves as a means of socially controlling women's lives, where men as individuals or as groups may exercise and maintain power over women and over other men via women's bodies. Individuals have to actively maintain and perpetuate their power over another. This takes place, as in the maintenance of any social order, by pressure to consent, including force, the threat of force and discursive pressures (Hester 1992: 1–2). While interpersonal violence and abuse are experienced materially and bodily, the impact may vary between individuals due to their location in particular sets of social relations and different contexts (Hester 2004). For instance, the impact of domestic violence on heterosexual men may be less severe than the impact on heterosexual women (Walby and Allen 2004), while the experiences of lesbians living in abusive relationships may be more heterogeneous than those of heterosexual women (Donovan and Hester 2007; Ristock 2002).

The relationship between gender, inequality and violence is of course something that is not straightforward, and is indeed contested. There has been a long and often heated debate in the Western academic literature regarding gender and interpersonal violence and abuse, with a questioning of the extent to which gender is an issue in the use and experience of violence and abuse. For instance, questions have been raised as to whether domestic violence is gender symmetrical – used equally by men and women in heterosexual relationships, or whether it is asymmetrical – with men and women using violence in different ways and with different consequences. However, the distinctions are often methodological, the product of using particular instruments, questions and samples (Archer 2000; Kimmel 2002). Similar debates have been evident in relation to child abuse, where questions have been raised about the extent of child sexual abuse, and gender of perpetrators (Farmer and Owen 2000; Russell and Bolen 2000).

To take one example, that of domestic violence, it can be seen that a reliance on a particular survey instrument in the United States and increasingly elsewhere, the Conflict Tactics Scale (CTS), has contributed largely to the notion that domestic violence might be gender symmetrical. Straus, Gelles, and Steinmetz (1980) developed the CTS in the attempt to provide replicable data on the incidence and prevalence of interpersonal violence. In its original format the CTS monitored how many times a man or woman had been violent towards their partner in the previous 12 months and how often the partner had been violent towards them in the same time period. The outcome of using this methodology led the researchers to conclude that heterosexual women and men were equally violent and that this type of interpersonal violence could be conceptualised as 'mutual combat' (Straus 1999). However, the emphasis on 'tactics' without contextual reference, and limitation of impact to physical injury (Straus 1999), has meant that studies using the CTS have often found it difficult to differentiate experiences of victimisation by men and women, where controlling behaviours may play an important part (Archer 2002). Moreover, the CTS approaches rely on and compare self-reports of perpetration by men and women as if these were indeed comparable. Yet evidence from qualitative research with women and men in heterosexual relationships indicates that answers to questions about abuse are gendered, with women tending to overstate, and men tending to underestimate, their violence against their partners (Hearn 1996; Miller 2001).

Heterosexuality, gender and inequality

Where 'sexuality' is concerned, both heterosexuality and same-sex contexts need to be taken into consideration. Not only is heterosexuality deemed the dominant sexuality – what may be termed 'hegemonic' – but within the idealised heterosexual context male and female sexualities are perceived and construed as different and unequal. MacKinnnon, for instance, referring to the construction of what is considered 'normal' heterosexuality, argues that 'male and female are created through the eroticization of submission and dominance' (1987: 136). Thus, men's power and women's social inferiority have become 'sexy'. The process of constructing women as erotic, or 'sexy', objectifies them, positioning women as subordinate and men as dominant. This process can be seen especially clearly within pornography (according to the Criminal Justice and Immigration Act 2008, an image is 'pornographic' if it has been produced for the purpose of sexual arousal), and it may be acted out more generally within heterosexual relations: where male sexuality objectifies the female object of desire, while female sexuality is objectified by the desired male subject (Hester 1992: 1).The huge growth in internet and video/DVD pornography (involving sexual exploitation of both adult women and children) and other forms of sexualised markets has helped to normalise the eroticisation of dominance, and thus also sanctioned gendered inequality and objectification of women (Itzin 2000a). For instance, in-depth research from the US (Frank 2003), where 30 men who frequented strip or lap dancing clubs were interviewed a number of times, found that over half of the men said that one of their motivations for visiting clubs was to escape the rules of conduct required when interacting with women in unregulated settings. The men found interactions with women more generally constraining. As one of the respondents said:

> You can go in there and shop for a piece of meat, quote unquote, so to speak. I mean, you want to see a girl run around naked. Have her come over, pay her to do a dance or two or three and walk away and not even ask her name. Total distancing.
>
> (Frank 2003: 66)

The normalisation and general availability of pornography, lap dancing clubs, etc., also creates a context where sexual violence becomes equated not only with gendered power, but more directly with male success. Bailey (2000) has pointed out that this may have detrimental consequences for vulnerable children and adolescents, such as the viewing of violent and pornographic videos by male adolescents who currently have no prospect of success in their own lives:

> Beyond the immediate content of violent and pornographic videos is the all too often spoken and unspoken message that violence and sexual assault are acceptable and related to individual success and satisfaction
>
> (Bailey 2000: 210)

In a further example, Messerschmidt (2005) explores how sexual violence as a 'masculine practice' enabled a teenage boy (Zack), who was bullied at school, feel good about himself. It made him feel 'dominant, powerful and heterosexual' (p. 208). Zack was bullied and beaten up by his male peers over a number of years for being fat. He ended up feeling 'pretty crappy about myself' (p. 206). In order to feel more like his peers, and to respond to the 'masculinity challenges' expected by them, 'he eventually turned to expressing control and power over his youngest female cousin through sex' (207). Over a period of three years he sexually assaulted his cousin 'by using a variety of seemingly nonviolent manipulative strategies' (207). Messerschmidt concludes, that while dominant meanings associated with masculinity helped to create a power divide between Zack and other boys at school, 'in the brief, illusory moment of each sexually violent incident – in which the sex offender practiced special and physical dominance over his cousin – Zack was a "cool guy"; the subordinate was now the dominant' (p. 208). Here the links between power and gender are seen in action, and how the acting out of a gendered male sexuality creates and re-creates gender inequality between Zack and his cousin.

To continue with the exploration of the importance of gender and sexuality to how violence and abuse 'work', and the normative practices associated with abuse, a further example, based on a compilation of women's experiences of sexual violence, will be outlined. The example illustrates in particular the processes of coercive control, as identified by Stark (2007), used in a context of gendered inequality, and especially the elements of entrapment. The process may also be seen as involving the 'grooming' otherwise associated with children being drawn into sexual abuse and exploitation.

> He asks her to dance. She accepts. (She wants to or she doesn't want to but she's afraid of hurting his feelings, she's afraid of making him angry, she wants a man to dance with.) He asks her out, she accepts. (She wants to, or she doesn't want to, but all her friends have got blokes, she's afraid of making him angry, he might feel hurt, she can't go out if she's on her own.) He kisses her. He puts his hand on her leg, her breast, her cunt. He wants to see how far he can go. She lets him. (She wants to or she doesn't want to but he's taken her out after all, and spent money on her, she needs a lift home, she doesn't want to seem a prude, he might be angry.) He asks her to sleep with him. She accepts. (She wants to, or she doesn't want to but she thinks she might as well, she can't back off now, it might be OK, she's flattered that he wants her, he might be angry.) Or she refuses. He tries to persuade her. He tells her he loves her. He says she doesn't love him. He calls her a prude, immature, frigid. He says he 'needs' sex, so if she won't come across, he'll have to find a girl who will. Each time they meet he carries on a bit further, a bit further. (Why not go all the way?) He buys durex to demonstrate his sense of responsibility. Each time she finally tells him to stop, breaks away, he gets angry, he rages, he sulks; he tells her how bad it is for men to be left 'excited'. (Prick-teaser!) He teaches her to suck him off. He works towards his goal, which is to have, to possess this woman.
>
> (London Rape Action Group, in Hester 1992: 65–6)

Within this script, both the man and the woman are active participants. However, their different and gendered positions means that it is the woman who gradually complies and becomes victimised. The action is geared towards the man. For the man the scenario appears to represent a normal heterosexual encounter. For the woman it is not so straightforward, and there is a tension between her apparent wish to become involved, and the encounter being intrusive and abusive. Indeed, this is a common rape scenario, where the woman is left confused because she is not sure that her feelings of violation and intrusion are correct, or whether it is the man's version (that the events are normal and merely what should have happened) is indeed correct. Again it can be seen how coercive control within a heterosexual context is linked to gender inequality – and draws on, creates and recreates such inequality.

Lesbians and gay men, inequality and gender

Much of the research on violence and abuse in relation to lesbians and gay men has been on the topic of 'hate crime', in other words, homophobic violence directed at the gay community by individuals or groups who want to undermine and threaten the very existence of lesbians and gays (Moran and Skeggs 2004). Such violence serves (as was seen in the case of gender) to reinforce inequality and discrimination against lesbians and gays. While such violence is not the focus of this volume, and will not be discussed further, it does highlight the unequal positioning of lesbians and gays in society, and the importance of considering inequality in any analysis of violence and abuse among lesbians and gays.

There is a small, although growing, body of knowledge about domestic violence in same-sex relationships (see Hester and Donovan 2009). There is an even smaller literature on sexual violence against lesbians and gays, and it is not always clear if the studies are including sexual violence by strangers as well as known individuals (Davenport et al. forthcoming). The discussion in this section will focus on the example provided by same-sex domestic violence.

Hester and Donovan (2009) outline how during the 1980s and 1990s there was some discussion, in the UK and elsewhere, about domestic violence in lesbian relationships and to a lesser extent gay male relationships, and how such behaviour might be tackled. At the same time, there were strong tendencies to minimise, hide, and deny the existence of such abuse. They highlight a number of factors that may be seen to have contributed to the greater invisibility of same-sex domestic abuse. These include fears of making obvious such problems within communities already considered 'problematic' in a homophobic society and contexts where conservative governments were attempting to reimpose 'traditional family values'.

The early literature and studies on same-sex domestic violence was focused mainly on lesbians (Hester and Donovan 2009). Lesbians were becoming visible as a domestic violence 'group', beginning to access domestic violence or rape support services ostensibly set up for heterosexual women or seeking help via lesbian or gay community organisations (Lobel, 1986). Studies on domestic violence in gay male relationships have emerged much more recently, building on concerns about and studies on gay men's health (Island and Letellier 1991).

Questions have been raised as to whether the 'gender and power' analyses of domestic violence, outlined in previous sections, can also be applied to domestic violence in same-sex relationships (Hester and Donovan 2009). Renzetti (1992), for instance, in research on lesbian domestic violence, argues that a gender and power analysis can be applied, but needs to be expanded to take into account the different experiences, meanings and interventions related to domestic violence that 'intersectionality' provides; that is, not just gender, but also the effects of location and discrimination linked to sexuality, race, and ethnicity. Ristock (2002) is more critical of the gender and power framework, seeing this as providing a heterosexual bias and wanting to focus on the specific experiences associated with lesbian domestic violence, while acknowledging the need to retain 'a necessary analysis of the pervasiveness of male violence against women' (ibid.: 20). By contrast, Island and Letellier (1991), focusing on gay men, argue that a 'gender and power' model does not apply at all to same-sex domestic violence and instead suggest that gender-neutral and individual psychological models should be applied. It has also been argued that violence in same-sex relationships are characterised by bi-directional 'common couple' or 'situational' violence, by contrast to heterosexual relationships where uni-directional 'patriarchal or intimate terrorism' is more prominent (Johnson 2006).

Studies from the US increasingly suggest that prevalence of domestic violence may be similar across same-sex and heterosexual relationships, and what differs are help-seeking behaviours (McClennen 2005). However, as Hester and Donovan (2009) point out, it is not possible to achieve random, representative samples of those in same-sex relationships and comparisons between studies on same-sex domestic violence are difficult because of the use of a variety of methodologies and samples, and varying definitions of violence and abuse. Consequently rates of prevalence have tended to vary enormously across the studies.

None the less it is possible to discern some patterns. The unequal positioning of lesbians and gays within society needs to be taken into account, as this has an effect on the forms of violence and abuse used within same-sex relationships, and also impacts on the extent to, and ways in which, lesbians and gay men seek help. At the same time, the processes of gender, identified above, also have an impact on the way violence and abuse 'work' in same-sex relationships, and on the resulting experiences and outcomes.

Age has been addressed in Part 2 of this volume: violence and abuse through the life-course. But it is also important here because both prevalence and general surveys indicate that age intersects with both gender and sexuality such that the use of and impacts of violence and abuse appear to be more intense for younger age groups, especially under 25s (Hester and Donovan 2009; Walby and Allen 2004).

Patterns of violence and abuse

This section will briefly explore some of the patterns of gender and sexuality that emerge from the wider studies on violence and abuse. For reasons of space, only a few, key, studies on domestic and sexual violence will be referred to. Echoing the debates earlier in this chapter, it will be seen that the overwhelming majority of those experiencing domestic or sexual violence are female, although a considerable number of men are also subject to domestic and/or sexual violence. What stands out, however, is that the vast majority of the abusers are heterosexual men, who victimise women and/or men.

Gender, domestic and sexual violence

Data on the prevalence of heterosexual domestic abuse in general populations show that both men and women may be violent against their partners. However, there are differences between men's and women's use and experiences of domestic violence, especially when frequency and impact are also taken into account. The national victimisation surveys from a number of countries, including the United States and United Kingdom (Povey et al. 2008; Slashinski et al. 2003; Tjaden and Thoennes 2000), suggest that while men and women in heterosexual relationships may use a similar range of domestic violence behaviours, there are also important differences. In particular, men administer a greater amount of and more severe abuse to their female partners than the other way round. Women are also more likely to use services, including health services and the police. The British Crime Survey (Povey et al. 2008) found that men tend not to report partner abuse to the police because they consider the incident 'too trivial or not worth reporting' (ibid.: 67).

Data from the 2005/06 British Crime Survey self-completion module on domestic violence, sexual assault and stalking (Coleman et al. 2007) found that women were more likely than men to have experienced partner abuse, family abuse, sexual assault and stalking since the age of 16. The differences between men and women were less marked in relation to experiences in the last year. It should be noted that the BCS figures outlined in this paragraph are based on CTS-type questions and relate to any one experience of the behaviours concerned (prevalence) and does not mean that the behaviours are necessarily part of an ongoing pattern. The authors of one of the BCS reports point out such prevalence tends to generate a spurious gender symmetry that vanishes if and when the impact of the act is brought into focus (Walby and Allen 2004: 37). The BCS found that since the age of 16, partner abuse (non-sexual) was experienced by 28 per cent of women and 17 per cent of men. Just under a quarter of women (23 per cent) reported having experienced stalking since age 16, and 13 per cent of men. Obscene or threatening phone calls or letters were the most common types of stalking behaviour experienced. Nearly half of the women (48 per cent) had experienced more than one type of intimate violence since age 16, while only a third (33 per cent) of men had experienced multiple forms. With specific regard to sexual violence, in the BCS survey just under a quarter (24 per cent) of women reported having experienced sexual assault since age 16, over half (54 per cent) from a partner or ex-partner, and altogether 89 per cent from known assailants. Most was less serious sexual assault (e.g. indecent exposure, sexual threats or touching, 23 per cent). Just under 6 per cent of women had experienced serious sexual assault and 5 per cent reported having been raped since age 16. The prevalence rates of sexual assaults were considerably lower among men (4 per cent any sexual assault and 1 per cent serious sexual assault), again mostly from known assailants (83 per cent).

However, the BCS also found that fewer men than women were impacted by the abuse or sought help for the consequences (Povey et al. 2008).[2] Men were less likely to report minor bruising or a black eye (16 per cent compared to 21 per cent) mental or emotional problems (14 per cent compared to 33 per cent); stopping trusting people (9 per cent compared to 15 per cent). Also, men were less likely than women to seek help from the police (9 per cent compared to 16 per cent) or seek medical help (18 per cent compared to 30 per cent). It should be noted that some of the male victims may have been in same-sex relationships, although the actual numbers are not known.

In the US National Violence Against Women (US NVAW) survey (Tjaden and Thoennes 2000) nearly 25 per cent of female respondents and 7.6 per cent of men surveyed said they experienced domestic violence (rape and/or physical assault) by a current or former spouse, cohabiting or dating partner at some time in their lifetime. The equivalent figures in the previous 12 months were 1.5 per cent of women and 0.9 per cent of men. Altogether, some 4.8 million intimate heterosexual partner rapes and physical assaults were found to be perpetrated annually against women in the US, and approximately 2.9 million intimate partner physical assaults against US men. The women were virtually all sexually assaulted by men, while most (70.1 per cent) of the men who were raped since the age of 18 were also raped by a male (Tjaden and Thoennes 2000: 47). Stalking by a current or former spouse, cohabiting partner, or date was also a key feature. Almost 5 per cent of women and 0.6 per cent of men reported being stalked some time in their lifetime, with 0.5 per cent of women and 0.2 per cent of men reporting being stalked in the previous 12 months. The authors conclude: 'These findings suggest that intimate partner violence is a serious criminal justice and public health concern' (Tjaden and Thoennes 2000: iii).

The US NVAW survey also found that women experience more chronic and injurious physical assaults at the hands of intimate partners than do men (ibid.: iv). Women averaged 6.9 physical assaults by the same partner, while men experienced on average 4.4 assaults. Also, 41.5 per cent of the women were injured during their most recent intimate partner assault, compared with 19.9 per cent of the men.

As a consequence of the more severe domestic violence and abuse that is used by men against their (usually female) partners, men are also the largest group to be recorded as domestic violence perpetrators by the police (Buzawa and Buzawa 2003; Hester 2006). This asymmetrical pattern of men as the main domestic violence perpetrators has been reflected in police records across many areas of England (Hester and Westmarland 2005; Hester 2006). In Northumbria, for instance, the vast majority of intimate partner violence perpetrators recorded by the police were men (92 per cent) and their victims mainly female (91 per cent) (Hester and Westmarland 2007).

Further differences have been highlighted in studies involving criminal justice and related samples. Hamberger and Guse (2002), for instance, in a criminal justice sample in the United States found that the men initiated significantly more violent episodes than did women and were more likely to start the overall pattern of relationship violence. The men reported less fear, anger, insult, and more amusement when their partners were violent than did women. In contrast, qualitative evidence from heterosexual relationships indicates that women are rarely the initiators of violence, are more likely to be acting in self-defence, and may be using a range of behaviours to do so (Downs et al. 2007; Miller and Meloy 2006; Saunders 2002). Johnson (2006) found that women, in particular, may use 'violent resistance' against violent male partners where men are 'intimate terrorists'. Miller and Meloy (2006), in a study of violent behaviour that led women to be arrested on domestic violence charges in the United States, conclude that 'the truly violent woman is an anomaly' (p.104). Instead:

> ... most women used violence to thwart their husbands' or boyfriends' egregious actions, to defend themselves or their children, or because their current situation mirrored earlier circumstances in their lives where they perceived or experienced danger and violence.
>
> (Miller and Meloy 2006: 104).

Research by Hester (2009) compared cases of domestic violence involving female or male victimisation recorded by the police. Directly comparable samples of cases with male perpetrators, female perpetrators or 'dual' perpetrators were established from police records and tracked over six years. The findings echo previous studies in showing that violent and abusive behaviour between heterosexual partners in contact with the police is gender asymmetrical. While cases were very varied, there were significant differences between male and female perpetrators of domestic violence in many respects. Men were the perpetrators in a much greater number of incidents;

the violence used by men against female partners was much more severe than that used by women against men; violence by men was most likely to involve fear by and control of female victims; women were more likely to use weapons, often in order to protect themselves. In addition, the police were more likely to describe female perpetrators as alcoholic, or mentally ill, although alcohol misuse by men had a greater impact on severity on outcomes. The research highlighted that men and women – both as victims – were using different approaches to managing their own safety, which were linked to their different, gendered, positions of power. The men were more able to take an active approach, removing themselves from the vicinity of the violent partners, removing weapons or imposing restraints. In contrast, women in fear of their partners had to negotiate safety by giving in to the demands of the violent men, in ways that appeared to further compromise their safety in the longer term.

Whether or not an individual is perceived as a perpetrator or a victim can be complex, and involves gendered perspectives and constructions by the professionals involved. In research on police interactions with domestic violence victims and suspects in the United States, DeLeon-Granados and Long (2000) observed how male domestic violence suspects were able to influence decisions made by officers at the scene of the crime using 'an often-subtle but powerful language' that 'conspired against female victims and helped male suspects to minimize their actions, deny responsibility, and shift blame' (ibid.: 361). The authors argue that 'Batterers work to manipulate the system not only to protect themselves from punishment but also as a way to maintain positions of power in their intimate relationships' (DeLeon-Granados et al. 2006). The types of gendered dynamics described by DeLeon-Granados and colleagues (2006) and Miller (2001), whereby men in criminal justice settings may minimise their actions and consequently the blame on themselves, or women may minimise their experiences of violence from male partners, were also echoed to some extent in the research by Hester (2009). For instance, men were able to minimise their own violence by not providing a statement to the police in some cases where their partners had used violence in retaliation or self-defence, and/or they had themselves been extremely violent. In contrast, women who were victimised, at times withdrew statements, minimised or denied that violence had taken place against them where male partners were also very threatening and controlling (Hester 2009).

Lesbian and gay domestic and sexual violence

The national US Violence Against Women survey (NVAW) (Tjaden et al. 1999; Tjaden and Thoennes 2000) included a small sub-sample of individuals identifying as gay or lesbian, and is one of the only representative studies to compare heterosexual and same-sex samples. It found that in same-sex relationships, male respondents were more likely than women to report violence from intimate partners; and that women in heterosexual relationships were the most likely to report violence (Tjaden et al. 1999). Of women living with a female intimate partner, slightly more than 11 per cent reported being raped, physically assaulted, and/or stalked by a female cohabitant – compared to 30.4 per cent of the women who had married or lived with a man as part of a couple and who reported such violence by a husband or male cohabitant. Approximately 15 per cent of the men who had lived with a man as a couple reported being raped, physically assaulted, and/or stalked by a male cohabitant, compared with 7.7 per cent per cent of the men who reported such violence by a wife or female cohabitant. Unfortunately, no measures of impact were explored regarding same-sex relationships. The authors suggest that more research is needed to support or refute whether these findings indicate that there is more domestic abuse in heterosexual contexts, although the evidence does indicate that intimate partner violence is generally perpetrated by men, whether against male or female intimate partners. They conclude as a consequence, that 'strategies for preventing intimate partner violence should focus on risks posed by men' (Tjaden and Thoennes 2000: v).

The most detailed study in the UK of domestic and sexual violence in same-sex relationships is that of Donovan and Hester (2007). This research engages with issues of both gender and sexuality, using a multi-method approach with a national community survey, focus groups and follow-up interviews. More than a third of the survey respondents (38.4 per cent) said that they had experienced domestic abuse at some time in a same-sex relationship, including similar proportions of women (40.1 per cent) and men (35.2 per cent). While the questionnaire sample was not random, these figures none the less suggest that domestic abuse is an issue for a considerable number of people in same-sex relationships in the UK. An even greater number of respondents indicated that they had experienced at least one form of abusive behaviour from their same-sex partners. Echoing other studies (e.g. Renzetti 1992; Ristock 2002; Walby and Allen 2004), emotional abuse appeared to be more widespread among them than physical and sexual abuse. However, respondents were more likely to identify physically and sexually abusive behaviours as 'domestic abuse'. Self-definition was most closely identified where individuals appeared to have experienced multiple forms of abuse (Hester et al. 2010).

Ristock (2002) emphasises the heterogeneity of domestic violence experiences in lesbian relationships. The Donovan and Hester (2007) survey data also indicated many similarities including the range of abusive behaviours experienced by gay men and lesbians and the impacts of such behaviour. Nonetheless, there were also important differences that appeared to reflect wider processes of gendering and gendered norms (Hester and Donovan 2009). Gay men were significantly more likely to use physically and sexually abusive behaviours (Chi-square sig. at $p<.05$). Sexual abuse was where the greatest gender differences occurred, with male respondents significantly more likely than women to be forced into sexual activity, be hurt during sex, have 'safe' words or boundaries disrespected, have requests for safer sex refused, and be threatened with sexual assault. When experience of potentially abusive behaviours and impact were taken into account together, sexual abuse stood out even more clearly as a risk factor for gay men (see Hester and Donovan 2009; Hester et al. 2010). Regarding impact of the violence and abuse experiences, lesbians were significantly more likely in the UK study to be affected by emotionally and sexually abusive behaviour. Lesbians were also much more likely to report that the abuse made them work harder so as 'to make their partner happy' or in order 'to stop making mistakes', that it had an impact on their children or their relationship with their children, or made them stop trusting people (Hester and Donovan 2009).

There were also important features where the form of the abuse was linked specifically to a context of inequality for lesbian and gays as a sexual minority. In particular it was found that first same-sex relationships can be an affirmation of identity that result in a confusion between the exhilaration associated with having come out with the exhilaration of falling in love, so that abusive behaviours are overlooked or minimised (Donovan and Hester 2008). This may be confounded by a lack of knowledge about what to expect in same-sex relationships (see also Ristock 2002). Lack of embeddedness in lesbian and gay communities and/or friendship networks may create barriers to support and make it easier for abuse to continue. Such lack of embeddedness, combined with concerns about being 'outed', may also create a context for abuse by the partner who does not want to be outed (Donovan and Hester 2008). Both survey respondents and interviewees also expressed the lack of help and support for lesbian and gays experiencing domestic violence, an issue echoed in more recent Home Office research (Hester et al. forthcoming).

Previous chapters in this volume have examined the life-course, including focus on children. Previous work has also identified 'age' as an important difference in perceptions and experiences of domestic violence and other abuse (Eriksson et al. 2005; and see Walby and Allen 2004). Age was again a significant feature in the UK same-sex domestic abuse study, and often more so than gender or sexuality. Most abusive experiences, whether emotional, physical or sexual, were reported by those individuals under 35 years and in particular in relation to 'first' same-sex relationships (Donovan and Hester 2008).

Implications for policy and practice

As indicated in the sections above, gender and sexuality are important considerations in understanding the nature of victimisation, the experiences and impacts of violence and abuse, for different individuals. Gender and sexuality (as well as other factors such as age and ethnicity) consequently have a bearing on service use, service need and help-seeking. Acknowledging and engaging with the specific experiences and needs of different groups and individuals, whether female, male, or lesbian, gay, bisexual and transgender (LGBT) are thus important, are issues with which practitioners and policy-makers need to engage, and require that the specific contexts of abuse for the individual concerned be understood.

Studies referred to above indicate some of the similarities as well as differences in help-seeking patterns between heterosexual and LGBT communities. To give an example regarding experiences of domestic violence: Both heterosexual and LGBT individuals appear to use friends/relatives/neighbours as their main focus for seeking help and support following violence and abuse from partners (Donovan and Hester 2007; Walby and Allen 2004). (While the BCS is not strictly a 'heterosexual' survey, the figures for same-sex respondents to the interpersonal violence module have been deemed too small for the data to be meaningful, and do not indicate help-seeking for this population (Smith et al. 2010)) However, heterosexual victims, and heterosexual women in particular, appear much more likely to contact the police than lesbians or gay men. For heterosexual victims, this was the second largest help-seeking category in the BCS (Walby and Allen 2004). In contrast, lesbians and gay men are more likely to use private counselling support (Donovan and Hester 2007), while the use of mental health services by BCS respondents appears to be very low (Walby and Allen 2004). These overall patterns reflect the increasing emphasis on criminal justice interventions in mainstream policy on domestic violence, but also the concerns of lesbians and gay men about potential homophobic reactions from statutory services and the 'private' rather than 'public' nature of their help seeking (Donovan and Hester 2007).

With regard to use of GPs or medical services, women in the BCS were more likely than men to contact GPs, while in Donovan and Hester's same-sex survey it was gay men who were more likely than lesbian women to contact GPs. These patterns reflect the impacts of both gender and sexuality. Heterosexual women in general access GPs more than heterosexual men (see Payne 2006), one reason for this being the reluctance of men to be perceived as 'weak' or not 'masculine'. For instance as expressed by a man who had experienced domestic violence from his female partner, he was 'a bit of a tough old bird, a bit stubborn, ... a typical man' (Daryl in Hester et al. forthcoming) and therefore reluctant to go to the doctor. At the same time, heterosexual men who experience (or perpetrate) domestic violence are seemingly more likely to access GPs than other services for support and intervention (Hester et al. 2006; Westmarland et al. 2004). In contrast, the emphasis on health needs of gay men due to concerns about HIV/AIDS has meant that gay men more readily access health services than do lesbian women.

These patterns may differ where other forms of violence and abuse are also taken into account. For instance, research comparing service use and service needs of heterosexual men and women, gay men and lesbian women in relation to domestic and sexual violence, found that sexual violence or childhood sexual abuse led more often than domestic violence to severe impacts on health and well-being (e.g. self-harm, suicidal feelings), with disclosure and help seeking especially difficult for gay men and lesbians due to concerns about homophobic reactions and lack of understanding by practitioners about sexual violence experienced by gay men and lesbians or the impacts of such abuse on sexuality, for instance, that gay men experienced sexual violence mainly from male partners, in some instances with fear of exposure to HIV/AIDS, while lesbians experienced sexual violence from female partners, male ex-partners or other men (Hester et al. forthcoming).

To reiterate, this chapter has indicated that understanding how gender inequalities and processes as well as constructions of sexuality influence and intersect with regard to how individuals may use, experience and embody violence and abuse is important: it allows comparison of similarities and differences across abusive lesbian, gay male or heterosexual relationships, and allows consideration of possibly different experiences and different needs for these groups of individuals with regard to health and mental health interventions.

Notes

1 Lesbian and gay tend to be the terms used most frequently by individuals identifying as non-heterosexual (McCarry et al. 2008), and are therefore used here. It should be noted that queer, homosexual or transgender are terms individuals also use to describe their identity.

2 This and the following information is based on the 2004/05 BCS survey, which are the most recent data available.

7 Race and culture

7.1 Asian and minority women, domestic violence and mental health The experience of Southall Black Sisters

Hannana Siddiqui and Meena Patel

The year 2009 marked the 30th anniversary of Southall Black Sisters (SBS), which was founded in 1979 to address the needs of Asian and African-Caribbean women. It provides advice and advocacy services, and campaigns and conducts policy work on gender-based violence in minority communities, particularly South Asian. Although based in Southall, West London, the work of SBS has a national reach due to its work on domestic violence, suicide and harmful cultural practices such as forced marriage and honour crimes, and related issues of racism, poverty, homelessness and immigration matters. Over the years, it has helped thousands of black and minority ethnic (BME), predominantly South Asian, women escape abuse within the family. Most of these women also report high levels of depression and self-harm. Indeed, most report having contemplated or attempted suicide at least once in their lives, and a tragic few have also actually committed suicide. These facts are even more horrific when placed in the context of the wider picture. Research shows that South Asian women are up to three times more likely to kill themselves than women in the general population (Raleigh 1996). They also have a disproportionate rate of self-harm, attempted suicide and suicide ideation (Husain et al. 2006).

South Asian women's experiences of abuse and mental illness

Women who come to SBS often report feeling mild to severe depression with low self-esteem and high levels of self-harm and suicide ideation. Some cases are complicated by a severe clinical disorder, but most do not have a diagnosed mental illness, although many are on medication for depression. However, while the SBS psychotherapist often diagnoses women as suffering from post-traumatic stress disorder (PTSD), there is an acknowledgement that the illness is rooted in social causes. Most women have experienced abusive practices within the family, including assault, imprisonment, harassment, rape and sexual abuse, emotional blackmail and coercion, demands for a dowry, forced marriage, abduction and attempted murder. In SBS's experience, women who commit suicide or are murdered in domestic homicides often have a history of domestic violence and mental health problems. For example, in the case of Banaz Mahmod, a 19-year-old Iraqi Kurd, who was murdered in a so-called 'honour killing' in 2007 by her father, uncle and men within her community for wanting to marry an 'unsuitable' boyfriend after leaving her abusive husband, had seen a psychiatrist about her problems prior to her death.

Other women have a number of issues or compounding factors, which may make their experience of abuse and mental illness even more acute. Those with an insecure immigration status, for instance, may also be fearful and anxious about the threat of deportation to their country of origin where they face problems of social ostracism, harassment and violence, especially as divorced, separated or single women. This is often the case for women who have separated from abusive spouses or partners in the UK or those claiming asylum on the grounds of gender-related persecution. Many with an insecure status are also anxious about having 'no recourse to public funds', which means they cannot claim most social security benefits or public housing. These women are unable to leave abusive relationships or are subjected to economic and sexual exploitation due to the experience or fear of destitution. These women have a stark choice: destitution or further violence.

Examples include that of 'Balwant' and 'Gurpreet' (both pseudonyms). Balwant is an 18-year-old Asian woman who escaped domestic violence and a forced marriage. Balwant married in India, and joined her British national husband in the UK in 2008. She was physically and sexually abused by her husband. She was also beaten and abused by her in-laws. Her mother-in-law, for instance, instigated her brother-in-law to rape her, and her sister-in-law attempted to burn her to death. Balwant also suffered a miscarriage and when her husband and in-laws attempted to abort her second child, a nurse helped Balwant to escape. Balwant was eventually referred to SBS for assistance. During her time with her husband and in-laws, Balwant took an overdose due to severe depression.

Twenty-two-year-old Gurpreet came to join her husband in Britain after marrying in India. She experienced abuse from her husband and her mother-in-law. Forced to sell her jewellery to pay her dowry, she was imprisoned in the house where her husband would frequently rape her. Her sister-in-law would also beat her and encouraged others to do so. Gurpreet felt she could not leave her husband because of her insecure immigration status, which also meant she could not claim benefits. She grew depressed and attempted suicide by cutting her wrists with a knife. She had contemplated setting herself alight several times before. After a beating, Gurpreet was sent to live with another family member, who abused her until she suffered injury. Gurpreet complained to her GP, who prescribed antidepressants, but also used the opportunity to refer her to SBS, where she was helped to leave home.

Some women also experience high levels of depression and self-harm in particular settings. Those in prison or detention centres, for instance, are particularly vulnerable, as highlighted by the case of Zoora Shah. In 1992,

Zoora Shah, a South Asian woman from Pakistan, was convicted of the murder of a man with whom she had a long-term relationship. He had subjected her to economic and sexual exploitation, including raping and pimping her to other men. The appeal against conviction was unsuccessful. The case highlighted the criminal justice system's failure to recognise her experience of domestic and sexual abuse, as well as the prostitution of women, within the Asian community.

In 2000, SBS successfully worked with lawyers to reduce her tariff from 20 to 12 years. SBS was instrumental in ensuring that Zoora was transferred to an open prison before obtaining parole in 2006. Prison support was provided by SBS. As the prison service had failed to provide regular counselling to help Zoora's rehabilitation, the SBS counsellor undertook intensive counselling to overcome trauma. Her counselling allowed her to express her regrets about her actions, which eventually showed the parole board she was fit to be released into the community.

No way out

Whenever confronted with the reality of suicide by a woman, the question is often asked as to why she felt that she had no option but to kill herself. Upon listening to women, however, it becomes apparent that the routes to escaping abuse for BME women are more limited than those for women more generally. They have greater barriers within and outside the community to overcome in order to access mainstream services and support, due to the failure of minority communities and the state to address their needs. Most policies and initiatives either ignore issues of race and gender or are specific to race or gender, neglecting the fact that BME women require interventions relevant to both their race and gender simultaneously. In other words, as BME women stand at the intersection of race and gender, their needs are often rendered invisible.

Within the community, strong social, religious and cultural pressures prevent BME women from leaving abusive situations. For South Asian, Middle Eastern and other minority women, for instance, cultural notions of sharam (shame) and izzat (honour) held by conservative sections of the community, often supported by orthodox religious beliefs, aim to control women's sexuality and autonomy, and act as powerful obstacles to women seeking help, leaving home or challenging abuse. Married women are expected to save their marriages at all costs and girls/young women are required to stay at home with their parents and families until married. They often face excessive restrictions on their lifestyles such as lack of freedom of dress, movement and association, or the right to pursue higher (or, in some cases, a basic) education and a career of their choice.

Failure to conform to traditional roles as an obedient and dutiful wife, daughter, sister, sister-in-law and daughter-in-law would bring shame and dishonour onto the extended family and the wider community. The consequence or 'punishment' for failing to do so often results in social ostracism or being 'disowned' and isolated, sexual harassment, threats to kill, assaults and even murder or a so-called 'honour killing'. This abuse or 'honour based violence' can be perpetrated by or involve the collusion of the whole extended family and community, including community and religious leaders. The words of Gurpreet express these pressures powerfully:

> My parents told me that I had to go back and make the marriage work. They were worried about how this would be seen in the community, and how they would be dishonoured by my very presence ... some people in the community put pressure on me to reconcile with my husband so that I would not continue to bring dishonour. When I have to tell people that I am divorced, no one asks why. They only assume that I must have been wrong, that it was my fault. They want me to die at home with my husband rather than leave him.

Women who suffer mental health problems as a consequence also experience stigma. Like most communities, mental illness is a taboo subject where families are often confused about how to treat the problem or are in denial, although some are supportive and refer women to a doctor for counselling or appropriate psychiatric treatment. For BME women, however, there are additional issues. South Asian women who refuse to conform to traditional expectations, such as those challenging abuse, can be labelled as being 'bad' or 'mad'. They are either 'punished' for being 'morally loose women' or receive 'treatment', which can include medication, hospitalisation and even electric shock treatment (which takes place overseas). Others are beaten, forced into marriage or abandoned.

The most extreme response is where there is a belief that the woman is possessed by demons and evil spirits. In this case, the family or community may turn to an unofficial 'witchdoctor' who uses black magic to heal her, or to the priest, who drives out evil spirits through prayer, and sometimes, even a beating. This led to tragic consequences in the case of Kousar Bashir. In 1992, a father and two Muslim clerics were involved in the torturing of 20-year-old Kousar Bashir to death during a ritual exorcism. The woman's father was convicted of murder having acted on the instructions of the clerics, who were found guilty of causing grievous bodily harm.

Multiculturalism to social cohesion and multi-faithism

Historically, the response of health and other agencies is perhaps best epitomised by Miriam Stoppard, who in the 1980s said that the state should not intervene to deal with mental health issues in relation to Asian women because such issues are resolved internally within the community. This 'multicultural' approach assumes that minority communities are self-governing and that the majority community must respect cultural difference in order to promote good community or race relations. To do otherwise would be intolerant and even racist. On these grounds, self-styled conservative and male community and religious leaders, regarded as the 'gate-keepers', refuse outside 'interference' on issues such as domestic violence. The failure of multiculturalism to recognise structural inequalities and power divisions within minority communities meant that the state colluded in the oppression of women by not intervening to protect women from gender-based violence. This represents a form of subtle racism because it discriminates against BME women by preventing them from accessing state support and protection.

In the last ten years, however, this multicultural or cultural relativist approach has come under attack. In 1999, the then Home Office Minister, Mike O'Brien, advocated a 'mature multiculturalism'. In the context of arguing for more state action to tackle forced marriage, he said that: 'multicultural sensitivities are no excuse for moral blindness'. He supported the SBS position that the state needed to intervene in order to uphold the rights of women within BME communities, while also recognising that minority cultures had some positive values and customs which should be respected. Since then, a greater willingness by government and other statutory agencies to address harmful cultural or traditional practices such as forced marriage, honour-based violence and female genital mutilation has been evident.

However, since 9/11 and 7/7, the gains of 'mature multiculturalism' were soon overshadowed by the new cohesion agenda, at the heart of which is the need to fight terrorism and Muslim extremism in particular. This has changed the nature of the state's relationship with minority communities from that of multiculturalism to that of 'assimilation', although this has been dressed up as 'integration'. Increasingly minority communities are expected to adopt 'core British values' based on the assumption that these values are inherently more liberal than those held by minority communities. And yet, paradoxically, government has also promoted 'multi-faithism', encouraging greater 'religious sensitivity' and funding for faith-based, particularly Muslim, initiatives. This has resulted in stronger conservative religious identities, which have placed women under pressure to stay within abusive situations through mediation and reconciliation by community elders or religious arbitration via Islamic Sharia courts. These serve to place abused women with mental health problems in a more vulnerable position, particularly where agencies also use religious institutions to provide 'therapy'.

Current interventions

This shift in policy from multiculturalism to 'multi-faithism' and social cohesion threatens the gains made by the BME women's movement, which, in the last thirty years, have established specialist refuge, advocacy and counselling services, and successfully campaigned for legal and social policy reform on violence against BME women. Indeed, progressive secular feminist organisations like SBS are threatened with closure as funding is diverted to religious and generic organisations in a context where local authorities attempt to cut costs and deliver on their social cohesion policies, conveniently using the argument that 'single group funding' is counterproductive to a cohesive society, despite legal rulings to the contrary.

These developments have dangerous consequences for BME women, who depend on specialist BME women's services to access both support within the community and mainstream services to escape domestic violence and overcome mental health problems. Community-based provision for specialist counselling or 'talking therapies' and BME women's refuge, advocacy and support services are already few and far between. Loss of funding for the BME women's sector will erode this further.

By comparison, there has also been little or no development within mainstream health services with regard to addressing the specific needs of BME women experiencing abuse. While there have been some Department of Health (DH) programmes such as the Victims of Violence and Abuse Prevention Programme (Itzin 2006) and Women's Mental Health into the Mainstream (DH 2002b), which recognise issues affecting BME women, their impact or implementation has been limited or nonexistent. The Delivering Race Equality programme (DH 2005a) promoted 'culturally competent' services, but these do not focus on the needs of BME women and uncritically allow for religious organisations to be part of the therapeutic intervention. Although the National Suicide Prevention Strategy (DH 2002a) recognises Asian women and suicide as an issue, it places strategies to tackle the problem in the lower goal 2 category, rather than in goal 1, which targets high-risk groups.

More recently, in 2008, the DH consulted on a Framework for Violence and Abuse Prevention (DH 2008), but this has been heavily criticised by women's groups for medicalising women's experience of abuse and ill-heath, and for supporting disputed 'cycles of abuse' theories. In late 2009, the DH also established a Violence Against Women Task Force. It is too early to state how effective this will be. There is also a concern that government funding has emphasised support for short-term cognitive behaviour therapies with little resources for other types, such as those which tackle PTSD, and longer-term interventions.

Using the courts

While SBS and others have or are using these initiatives to influence change, SBS has also uniquely used the Coroner's courts to increase state accountability in domestic violence and suicide cases with the aim of preventing future fatalities. Over the years, SBS has dealt with 17 suicides or death by unknown causes. In 13 of these, SBS assisted the family or friends of the deceased to raise the possibility at the Inquest that domestic violence may have contributed to the death, and in so finding, the Coroner should make recommendations to agencies on improvements in policy and practice to address the problem. Coroners often resist examining the history of domestic violence, and limit their inquiry to the immediate circumstances, and to 'how', 'when' and 'where' rather than 'why' the death took place.

While in some cases, with legal representation, the Coroner has been persuaded to explore the issue of domestic violence, sometimes accepting expert evidence from SBS on cultural and religious pressures on Asian women experiencing abuse, none has been willing to attribute a suicide directly to domestic violence or find shortcomings in the response of agencies involved in the case. Often their attitude has been dismissive. In one case where an Asian woman jumped onto a railway line with two of her small children, the Coroner's courts ignored the history of abuse, even though the woman was known to the mental health services for being depressed about her home circumstances. The serious case review into the children's deaths also ignored these issues. In another case, where an Asian woman died of unknown causes after experiencing domestic violence, the attitude of the Coroner, and the police officer who had been asked to investigate the case, was that of disbelief. The police officers stated that 'Asian women were less likely to regard forced sex in marriage as rape' and the Coroner concluded there was no evidence of domestic violence despite previous reports made to the police by the deceased herself!

In 2006, SBS also advised the Crown Prosecution Service in the case of *Dhaliwal*, which raised the issue of criminal liability for suicide as a result of domestic violence. The matter did not proceed to trial, as the courts ruled that there was insufficient evidence of psychiatric harm. This led SBS to call for a new law on criminal liability for suicide.

The SBS model of intervention

In 2001, SBS set up a domestic violence and mental health project for BME women. The project was a culmination of years of work on addressing these issues, particularly in relation to South Asian women. The project aimed to develop new models of intervention to reduce the incidence of domestic violence and mental health problems, suicide and self-harm among BME women. SBS developed a unique model that provided specialist holistic advice and advocacy services, which included information, advice, advocacy, befriending and one-to-one and group support services combined with psychotherapeutic-based counselling. These services provided for the needs of BME women, catering for their linguistic needs with an understanding of the dynamics of abuse within the context of their race, gender, religion and culture. The advice and advocacy services involved helping BME women with crisis to long-term casework assistance and support to enable them to escape violence and abuse, the befriending and support services helped to deal with intense loneliness and develop new skills, and counselling helped them to overcome depression and trauma. Ultimately, women were assisted to rebuild their lives enabling them to become independent, free from domestic violence and mental illness. This type of intervention came to be known as 'the SBS model'.

The project produced an action-based research report, *Safe and Sane*, which evaluated the project showing a high success rate (SBS forthcoming). These included the following outcomes: 70 per cent in a sample of 58 women assisted over six years had successful outcomes indicating they were better protected from abuse with lower levels of depression (only 6 per cent were unsuccessful; other outcomes were pending or unknown); for those in receipt of counselling, the success rate was 94 per cent with reduced reliance on medication and levels of self-harm. As part of the project, the SBS psychotherapist, Shahrukh Hussain, developed a new counselling 'hybrid model' which specifically catered for the needs of BME women experiencing abuse and combines humanistic, psychodynamic and life coaching approaches. A sample of service users expressed a 90 per cent satisfaction with the overall project, which they regarded as a 'home from home'.

The way forward

On the basis of the findings of the research, SBS recommends that fully funded holistic BME women's voluntary sector services based on the SBS Model should be replicated in every Primary Care Trust area with a high BME population.

Most BME women experiencing depression as a result of abuse are often prescribed medication. The 'medicalisation' of these problems by the health service therefore ignores the need to address the underlying social cause of mental illness. It is therefore recommended that statutory health and social care bodies should improve their response to BME women experiencing domestic violence and mental health problems by intervening to protect them from abuse and providing them with or referring them to appropriate advocacy and mental health services which operate within an equalities and human rights framework.

It is also recommended that the hybrid model should be adopted by mental health and counselling services. In particular, issues such as 'shame' and 'honour' and the impact of religion and culture on BME women experiencing domestic violence and harmful cultural practices should be officially recognised as a sub-category of post-traumatic stress disorder within the DSM-IV diagnostic criteria. More affordable or free counselling and 'talking' therapy services, as well as longer-term interventions are also required.

Other recommendations include the reforming of the Coroner's system to address suicide resulting from domestic violence and of the law to recognise criminal liability for suicide. Hospital and medical services should also ensure that women in their care are protected from abusive family and community members, particularly if they are incapacitated or unconscious as a result of physical and mental injuries sustained in suspicious circumstances, and that there is routine screening of domestic violence by all health departments, including by GPs and Accident and Emergency. Systems of confidentiality also need to be improved, particularly among family GPs and interpreters, and mandatory training and occupational standards would help to implement best practice. Institutionalised racism should also be addressed, for example, by providing specialist counselling and support to BME women in prison, detention centres and health services.

In addition, it is recommended that the DH establish an interdepartmental Ministerial Working Group to address domestic violence and mental health problems for BME women, with an initial task of conducting a public inquiry into suicide and self-harm. Government should also raise awareness and tackle attitudes and practices which condone domestic violence and challenge the stigma of mental illness within BME communities. Other new, such as the national violence against women strategy, and mainstream DH initiatives should integrate these issues, with a greater recognition of intersectional discrimination based on race and gender and an emphasis on successful implementation.

With reference to the general context, it is argued that social cohesion, multi-faithism, old style multiculturalism or cultural relativism and racist or discriminatory policies and practices do not protect BME women from domestic violence or help them overcome trauma, suicide and self-harm. Policies and practices based on mature multiculturalism, secularism, equalities and human rights are the only guarantors of BME women's freedom from domestic violence and mental illness.

7.2 Violence, agencies and South Asian women

Jalna Hanmer

I don't feel English people in particular understand what an Asian girl has to go through because it is different for them. It is very much different for them and when we tell them about all the beatings we've had, and everything, they say: 'Why don't you do this, why don't you do that'. It's the law in Britain, nobody can touch you. I don't think they understand at all.

(Interview with South Asian woman)

What is it that agencies fail to understand? Interviews in the North of England were held with women either from South Asia or whose families were. Given the population distribution, the majority of the 30 interviews were with women from or with family backgrounds in Pakistan. Interviews were conducted in English, Urdu and Punjabi. With women's permission, the agencies women approached were then contacted for interview. A brief description of a research approach on how agencies responded to South Asian women is followed by discussion of issues of communication and help seeking based on women's experiences of health and other agencies. Some of the major socio-cultural differences between girls and women who have lived in West Yorkshire for years and more recent migrants from South East Asia are interspersed throughout.

Mapping pathways: phases and clusters

Research into mapping pathways illuminates the various ways in which knowledge of South East Asian women's lives are lacking and limitations in the responses of agency staff stemming from their organisations and remits. Mapping pathways explored in depth how agencies network and cooperate with each other when responding to requests for help from women with personal or family backgrounds from South East Asia. There were no standard situations or agencies involvement in the 30 interviews.

Pathways were composed of varied experiences of violence, victimisation and agencies that became involved. Diagramming sequential mapping of agency contacts described progress from the first to subsequent agencies in the pursuit of help seeking. If referrals from one agency to another led to non-resolution of a woman's problem, later on she would begin again with another agency and its referrals. Phases continued until women's attempts to find ways to restrict and finally to remove themselves and their children from a violent household were successful. Multiple phases were commonplace, occurring over a number of years. One half of the women interviewed had one perpetrator, which could include one man only and, in extended households, his relatives.

The other one half experienced clusters of violence. Clusters occurred when women experienced violence from more than one perpetrator, for example sexual and physical violence begun in childhood and, later on, extended into their marriages or to other men known to the women, including family friends and more remote relatives. Alternatively, violence with a single perpetrator, which could include his family, could expand to her children or her mother, or other family members. In mapping pathways each different perpetrator and victim was identified as a separate cluster as help seeking involved different combinations of agencies. Clusters were experienced sequentially or, if one or more were not resolved before another began, cumulatively. Clusters of violence also had phases.

The decision to leave was more often than not made slowly and, without agencies available to help girls and women, there would be no escape. Agencies almost always offered some assistance, however inadequate. Responses from health agencies illustrate problems in communication, referrals and networking with other agencies.

Mapping help seeking and health agency responses

Major issues reducing the effectiveness of health agencies were inadequate attention to obtaining disclosures, with incorrect referrals associated with lack of disclosure, restricted networks of agencies, lack of contact between the agencies women were in contact with and not focusing on the problem which included more than the woman's experience. Both women and agencies experienced communication problems with each other. The limited remits of different agencies were neither understood nor important to women because their experience of violence and the needs it raised were unified. The experience of violence seamlessly affected her, her children, her residence, her income, her safety.

Professionals in General Practice, hospitals and mental health might realise a woman was experiencing a non-medical problem, but be unable to obtain disclosure. Women with children all attended General Practice surgeries or health centres and hospitals for the birth of children. Hospital staff could pay attention to unusual behaviour, such as the woman's husband rarely or never visiting his wife, showing no interest in the child, and she could be tearful. Hospital staff did ask, 'why are you crying?' and 'where is your husband?', but these efforts did not result in disclosure. Women who did not speak English were particularly disadvantaged. Unable to communicate with staff, their husband's family had additional control over women's non-disclosure of ill treatment. For women who could speak some English, her in-laws could be exceptionally kind and caring while she was in hospital to ensure her silence.

Women also attended hospital for self-harming, attempting suicide and, when not intending to do so, by overdosing. These conditions could result in being referred to or being seen by the psychiatric services before discharge, again, without disclosure. Women were medicated and in mental health units for short periods of time over years. The possible connections between these outcomes with domestic violence were not pursued.

Disclosure could happen because a woman's injuries were so extreme, but even then there could be no further action other than attending a hospital accident and emergency department. The opposite outcome also happened. One seriously injured woman, with injuries so obvious that too many people in the neighbourhood knew about it, went to her General Practice surgery where the doctor called the police. Involving other agencies was not always without danger as later this doctor was threatened by the husband's family. On occasion referrals could be inappropriate or the reason for the referral misunderstood. One doctor was reported as referring a woman to a psychiatrist in order, she thought, to assist her with an application for housing. This referral led to numerous mental hospital admissions.

There could be little or no contact between agencies and each agency had its own restricted network. Health had very limited networks that consisted largely of different forms of the organisation of health services. When health played a central role in a woman's life it could be even easier for other agencies to ignore the family perpetrators of the violence. Women were identified as having the problem, rather than others being identified as causing the problem.

The issues affecting the ability and willingness of women to communicate with agencies were complex. Women could rarely leave their extended family homes and there might be no one within who would provide information on sources of help. They were escorted to agencies, such as primary care, and to hospital, where oversight of their communication with professional staff was closely monitored. Women might believe or have been told that statutory agencies could not or would not intervene to assist. This response to women from other family members had some validity as agency non-intervention ranged from a refusal to intervene at all to not assisting women to disclose their distress. Women's attempts to communicate with agencies were not always successful. There could be non-intervention, a lack of interest in relevant earlier violent life experiences, and interventions that did not help.

What do agencies need to know?

It is of central importance to agency practice to recognise that marriage to other family members intensifies connections between the individual, the family and the community. Arranged marriages to non-family loosen this connection (non-family members are marriage partners for women from Sikh and Hindu religious backgrounds) with freely chosen marriage partners the most weakly linked. Muslim girls from Pakistan are both married to family relatives, preferably to first cousins on their father's side, and to non-family although this is less socially desirable. Attempts to separate or divorce when women are married to family members ruptures more than the marriage; both the wider family and community are deeply involved and affected. For effective intervention, agencies need understanding of the major socio-cultural factors that influence the possibilities for change open to individual women.

Whether from the UK or Pakistan, women's experiences of violence were centred on psychological, sexual, physical, financial and controlling behaviours, which could involve both themselves and their children (Hanmer 2000). Both women born in the UK and from other countries lived in multi-occupied housing with their in-laws and other family members, which increased the likelihood of violence from family members in addition to their husbands.

Understanding and accepting women's rights and role in arranged marriages and in married life differed between women who were brought from Pakistan for marriage and women who spent their childhoods in England. Those brought into England for marriage, both educated and illiterate and from different social classes, experienced little or less conflict about the position and expectations of women prior to and after marriage. Women from Pakistan described the community belief that husbands in relation to wives was: 'He is her God'. The role of a good wife, one that brings honour on her, and on her and his family, is circumscribed. She cooks, cleans, stays at home and looks after the children and obeys her husband and in-laws.

Girls could be married very young. UK-based girls were married in Pakistan prior to 16 years and often left with his family until they became pregnant when they were allowed to return to the UK. The youngest interviewed woman was married aged 13 in Pakistan and, as is usual, later married in England when the age of marriage was reached. Marriages could be arranged for young children, although women were unaware of the arrangements until adult or nearing adulthood. The responses and needs of women differed markedly with their country of origin, immigration status, age and knowledge of English being important factors.

Women's and men's experiences of unwanted marriages

Women born in the UK to parents from South Asia were less accepting of arranged marriages, both with family plans for and, when married without their consent, after their marriage. They experienced conflicts around women's autonomy to refuse a proposed marriage partner, to continue in employment or education, to control their own earnings and savings, to visit friends, some of whom could be from a different religion and culture. Young women could want more control over their lives. They had established relationships with boys, men, girls and women from the same and different cultural and religious groups, which their families regarded as unsuitable and attempted to end. One young woman said, 'I know quite a few girls at Asian and Black women's refuges that weren't escaping violence, they just wanted freedom'. As a result young women could move from city to city and refuge to refuge in an attempt to evade their families.

Once married and with her husband's arrival in England his community and family status was assured. His standing was not affected by a command of English or employable skills or employment or by the demands he made on his wife. She could be well integrated into British society, but once married she could be forced by her husband to leave work or education, he could take her savings, salary, and any other money that she received, beat and sexually abuse her, and require that she remained in the home. As the marriage deteriorated her family could try to intervene on her behalf but their actions were checked by the high status of the husband. When they advised her to follow the wishes of her husband and gradually ceased to intervene, when women had other supporters both friends, neighbours and employers who tried unsuccessfully to help, this was when women turned to agencies for assistance. Knowing English and more about the agencies available to help increased her ability to seek earlier intervention.

Both men and women with family backgrounds from South Asia were forced into marriage, but their response to a forced marriage differed greatly. Men could have ongoing relationships with English women that wives from South Asia knew nothing about. Once in England the husband could treat his wife as a servant, beat her and use her sexually as he pleased, ignore his children by her, refuse to financially provide for her and the children, take her dowry, both money and jewellery, while continuing his relationship(s) with other women. Families did criticise his behaviour but interventions by his, and her family if she had other relations in the UK, could be ineffective and over time gradually cease. This was when, often after years, women from South Asia turned to agencies for assistance.

Why is it difficult to leave?

When disclosure occurred, the advice to leave was given by all agencies, but this was often not followed. The question is why?

The major reason women found it difficult to leave was the concept of family honour, which rested on a woman's behaviour as a wife and affected both her family of origin and that of her in-laws. Leaving also could be forced on a woman rejected by the husband's family who could seek to retain her children while sending her back to Pakistan. Women desperately wanted to return to the marriage and were bewildered as they had fulfilled the requirements of a good Muslim wife. Women worried about harming their families of origin by adversely affecting their standing within South Asian communities. Women's options were severely curtailed as it was not possible for any of the interviewed foreign-born women to return to their country of origin. Some feared personal harm from the families of their in-laws if they returned, while others feared the dishonour that would be transferred to them and their family by the community.

Another major factor was his control over her. When there was an expectation from family and community that the relationship should continue, additional pressure was placed on women. In Muslim families from South Asia, authority over women passes from her family to his. As well as the husband, the father-in-law, if alive, and if not, the oldest son, are the primary sources of control over her behaviour. Her family may allow her to return for short periods, but her father, if alive, and if not, her eldest brother, determine how long she can stay before being returned to her husband and his family. The concept of family honour governs a woman's rights and role in arranged marriages and in married life. Honour affected values, beliefs and attitudes that circumscribed the behaviour of all the interviewed women and formed the background for marriage relations. This greatly increased his control over her and, with violence, her fear of him. As one well-educated woman from the UK expressed it, 'I never looked at him straight in the eyes. I would always gaze at his feet'.

Divorce was rarely a way out of a violent relationship. Without family permission to reject a marriage, women could be pursued relentlessly by their families. When divorce was seen as seriously harming the reputation held by the community of other family members, both his and hers, it could be avoided for many years, however he behaved. He could be an alcoholic, a drug addict, a gambler, have mental problems, known by his family and, possibly hers, to have been out of control from childhood as well as being directly abusive to her and their children. Some women described how the most they could hope for was permission from his and her family to live separately from their husbands, while others gradually gained family support to leave and to divorce. A divorce in England did not always solve the problem for some women as her husband could then refuse to give her a Muslim divorce. Separating without divorce verged on the impossible when he did not want this to happen.

Issues hindering positive outcomes

The advice offered to women by statutory agencies seemed to stem from an underlying assumption that women were free to make choices about their futures unhindered by family and other community members. The expectations and the exercise of control through families and communities were an essential part of the violence experienced which, if unheeded, affected women's abilities to take positive action to overcome the problems they faced and to effectively communicate with agency staff. Agencies were faced both with women trapped within violent marriages and women experiencing violence that were rejected from the marital home and wished to return.

Positive outcomes required action based on the principle that women and children were entitled to violence-free lives, but given agency procedures, practices and requirements, that could become an abstract, meaningless concept. There could be a lack of focus on the perpetrators of violence, even occasionally within criminal justice agencies. Among other statutory agencies a focus solely on the woman or the child was a common response even though perpetrators harassed and stalked women, had mental health and behavioural problems that made a non-violent home impossible to achieve. The perpetrator disappeared from view and could be seen as not relevant to the agency purpose. Non-engagement with perpetrators skewed the assessment of the problem by limiting it to fit in with agency practice.

There were multiple problems in agencies communication with women. It was more than not understanding the woman's context in which the problem was located, although very relevant and important. Nor was it solely a question of skills and training, although very relevant and important. Professionals were influenced by organisational factors, both formal and informal. Policies and procedures skewed understanding and interventions in particular ways which influenced women's abilities to communicate with agency staff as well as agency staff's ability to communicate with women.

Agencies were likely to decontextualise women's experiences of violence. There were three major issues. First, specific agency remits could disregard the overall impact of violence on women's lives. Mapping revealed unconnected clusters of agencies in relation to different perpetrators. These agencies were unlikely to know about prior violent events and different perpetrators even when they remained current issues for women. Secondly, women's experiences included repetition of violence, but prior incidents might not be considered as relevant or down-played when agencies responded. Thirdly, within any one agency system there could be a lack of relationship and connections within it. Record keeping could be poor or non-existent so when the worker who responded to a woman left, there could be no one remaining with knowledge of her.

Not fully exploring the problem, how women felt about it, what they tried to do about it, what they wanted as an outcome created further communication problems. Agency staff communication could rest on an imperfect understanding of what violence meant in the life of women and their children. Tolerating the adverse effects of violence to women and their children or being seen as some other agency's responsibility could be the result. Agency staff could visit women regularly without any improvement in their situations. There could be a lack of knowledge of risk factors that could assist in identifying women experiencing financial, physical, sexual and psychological abuse.

Networking

Networking among agencies is being promoted as a way to overcome these outcomes, while at the same time retaining restricted agency responses that do not, on their own, meet women's needs. A lack of knowledge of how other agencies could assist in achieving effective actions restricted referrals. When there was no working relationship with the referred to agency, knowledge of how they fitted into resolving the woman's problem could be limited and adversely affect the outcome. Inadequacy or even a refusal to help could be the result. When this occurred women had to begin again with another agency. The responsibility for explaining the problem and the help that was needed was thrown back onto women.

While effective multi-agency responses were difficult to achieve, women did experience effective working together by agencies. When this happened women could credit agencies, particularly the police, for saving their lives. Effective agency cooperation was more than relevant referrals. Working together successfully involved knowing which other agencies need to be involved and gaining their cooperation. Effective intervention by one specialist agency could impinge positively on the work of another contributing to successful individual agency and multi-agency work. Multi-agency responses became even more complicated when women experienced clusters of violent experiences. When the current issue was treated as the only problem in women's lives, it obscured the interconnections between each violent cluster and its phases weakening the abilities of agencies to provide effective interventions. The reason this was so relevant for individual women was that connections between violent clusters were central to their lives.

Agencies that worked solely on violence to women were another way of organising multi-agency interventions as they made referrals to the statutory agencies which women needed to resolve their domestic issues. Referrals to refuges were the most successful in meeting women's needs as their networks contained contacts with the specific multiple services of protection, housing, health, and income. Successful outcomes could occur when the civil and criminal justice systems focused on the perpetrator and other agencies provided assistance to women and their children or when they worked together to resolve an issue involving a perpetrator. When agencies had a close working relationship with each other, women were more likely to be effectively assisted. Women's Aid and Black and Asian refuges were likely to have good working relationships with specific solicitors, housing associations and local authority housing departments, domestic violence police units, and other professionals. Led by the requests of women, professionals collectively assisted women in freeing themselves from abusive men and their families.

Referrals were not the sole responsibility of agencies as women also referred themselves. Young women who came to the UK for marriage who spoke English were less disadvantaged than those who did not, but both were even less likely to know what services were available than girls and women from the UK. To organise their own multi-agency pathway, a woman needed a thorough knowledge of agencies in order to efficiently select those that could help with specific aspects of her and her children's problems. This knowledge could take years to obtain. In practice, pathways consisted of self-referral and agencies' referrals to each other in limited and sometimes in haphazard ways.

Improving practice

Responding to domestic violence against women is an extremely demanding area of practice. It places organisational demands upon agencies as well as demands for good practice on individual workers. For successful intervention, individual workers require knowledge of domestic violence, an in-depth understanding of specific women's problems and the social context in which a woman is located, the remits and abilities of other local agencies, previous agency contacts and interventions with women, and the totality of which agencies need to be involved. In order for individual workers to be effective the agency in which they are located needs policies and procedures that support intervention. These include specific training for workers, the allocation of sufficient time for workers to engage with the problem and network with other agencies, good record keeping, and ongoing evaluation of agency successes and failures. Agencies do not always have the financial resources and staff they need to be able to achieve these good practice requirements.

Improving practice and implementing good practice guidance will be aided by individual agency and multi-agency assessments of effective strategies and interventions. Systematic ongoing evaluation of inputs and outcomes can reveal problem areas within and between agencies in need of attention. If followed up by sufficient resources for problem solving and its evaluation, overall financial expenditure on this area of work can be reduced or more women and children can be helped. The sooner a problem can be resolved, the less it costs, in terms of both finances and personal suffering. Understanding and using pathway analysis created by self-referral and by agency referrals to each other has an important contribution to make to good practice and successful individual agency and multi-agency interventions.

8 Violence, abuse and disabled people

8.1 Learning-disabled adults and children

Richard Curen and Valerie Sinason

Introduction

Some of the key points that came out of the VVAPP programme were that disabled children and adults are more likely to be abused and that their abuse is less likely to be picked up. Also abuse can itself cause disabilities and accessing post-abuse support is often harder than for victims without disabilities. This chapter attempts to explore why this is so and what can be done about these serious problems. However, it is important to point out that anyone attempting to discuss matters such as these has also to address complex issues around difference (Haque 2009; Marks 2000), inequality (Herrington et al. 2007), loss (Bicknell 1983; Blackman 2003; Hollins 1999; Hollins and Grimer 1988), history (O'Driscoll 2009) and language (Sinason 1992a). No human group has been forced to change its name so frequently. What is obviously at work is a process of euphemism. Euphemisms are a verbal attempt to deal with taboo subjects, subjects that cause social disquiet. 'Intellectual Disability' is the now the main term used within Europe, and British groups are beginning to adopt this too (Cottis 2009), although in our opinions this term also fails to do justice to the wide spectrum of individuals it attempts to unite.

Traumatic external stressors in the origins of environmentally determined learning disability

The external stressors that lead to the majority of mild learning disability in the UK (Ricks 1990), such as lowest social class, poverty (Rieser and Mason 1992) largest number of siblings, paternal unemployment, maternal deprivation (Rutter et al. 1970) are clearly documented. The Office of Population Censuses and Surveys (UK) (OPCS) Study of Disabled Children (Bone and Meltzer 1989) found that boarding or alternative provision was needed for 48 per cent of disabled children who were at physical or emotional risk in their home environment (Marchant 2008).

The Interim Findings of the National Commission on Children, published in Washington on 28 April 1990 estimated that malnutrition affects

500,000 children in the USA, directly creating an illiterate underclass. An estimated 100,000 children are homeless. When it comes to organic learning disability, 300,000 severely learning-disabled children and adults live in the UK on average (Ricks 1990) and over 1 million children and adults have a mild learning disability, of whom the majority live in deprived circumstances (Rutter et al. 1970). Many have coexisting physical disabilities and, not surprisingly given the burden they carry, there is an increase in emotional disturbance in proportion to the severity of the handicap (McQueen et al. 2008).

This combination of inequality and inevitable trauma often leads, unsurprisingly, to heightened levels of abuse and domestic violence.

Attachment, loss and trauma

Childhood attachment is a prerequisite for safety. Spitz (1953) showed how children in an orphanage who were physically cared for but who had no attachment figures appeared learning disabled. In other words, the trauma of separation and loss in infancy can 'take the form of a retardation dependent on the severity and duration of the trauma' (ibid.: 35).

While separation can cause vulnerability for the child, being at home with an unresourced family can create further vulnerability too. Frodi (1981), Morgan (1987) and Herrenkohl and colleagues (1983) are among the many researchers who have found the stress a disabled baby evokes in a family, and the extra physical and emotional demands, triggers parental stress and abuse.

There is a recurring chicken and egg problem as to whether physical or learning disability causes the abuse as a stress factor in a family (Birrell and Birrell 1968) or whether the abuse caused the learning disability (Buchanan and Oliver 1979; Sinason 1992a). Ammerman and colleagues (1988) and Sullivan and Knutson (1998; 2000) examined the predisposing factors that led to increased risk of abuse and neglect of multiply handicapped children. They included disruption in mother–infant attachment, greater stress related to care needs and difficult behaviour problems, and increased vulnerability due to communication and/or cognitive limitations.

Sexual abuse of children and adults

Whilst the literature from the 1970s onwards (e.g., Lynch 1975; Sullivan and Knutson 1998, 2000; Sullivan 2003) has pointed to extra vulnerability to abuse of physically handicapped and learning-disabled children, there are very large gaps in epidemiological knowledge.

When a British psychiatrist (Cooke 1990), aware of the little attention given to the sexual abuse of learning-disabled adults in the UK, attempted to undertake a survey by sending questionnaires to a representative sample of learning disability consultants, she found a 4–5 per cent average prevalence rate, which her respondents found to hide a much higher hidden prevalence. Hard and Plumb (1987) in interviewing the total population of one day centre in America found 83 per cent of the women and 32 per cent of the men reported sexual abuse. However, these statistics leave open the question of how representative the samples are.

In the absence of accurate national and international figures the facts that come from admittedly biased samples are nevertheless worth noting. A sample of 201 children and adults with a learning disability referred to a North London outpatient psychotherapy service revealed an abuse level of 78 per cent in child referrals and 90 per cent of adults referred for aggression turned out to have been sexually abused (Sinason 2004).

Some researchers estimate that more than 90 per cent of people with developmental disabilities will experience sexual abuse at some point in their lives and 49 per cent will experience 10 or more abusive incidents (Valenti-Hein and Schwartz 1995)

In 2000 the Department of Health published 'No Secrets' (DH and HO 2000) which provides guidance to local agencies who have a responsibility to investigate and take action when a vulnerable adult is believed to be suffering abuse. Significantly the guidance did not offer the same legislative structure that Child Protection is afforded. It is hoped by many that the eagerly awaited publication of the review of the guidance will address this issue.

Physical abuse of children and adults

Sternfeld (1977) considered that 12.5 per cent of new cases of cerebral palsy each year in the US were caused by abuse, whilst in England Buchanan and Oliver (1979) found 3–11 per cent of their study were learning disabled due to violence and they coined the term VIMH – Violence Induced Mental Handicap. In addition, they reported that 22 per cent in residential institutions had been physically abused. In 1983 Akuffo and Sylvester (1983) examined 1400 accident forms and post-mortem records, concluding that injury from shaking or battering contributes significantly to learning disability. In 1988, Oliver studied 294 children and found 11 cases of VIMH. They also had epilepsy and other problems after abuse and neglect. He commented, 'Ill treatment in the home accounts for such conditions (learning disabilities) in 5 per cent or more of all handicapped people' (Oliver 1988). Diamond and Jaudes (1983) considered that at least 9.3 per cent of their sample became cerebral palsied as a result of physical abuse. Cohen and Warren (1987) point out that physical abuse figures for acquired disability are higher than for those where the disability was present at birth.

Acts of abuse by learning-disabled parents

Parents who are learning disabled are more likely to be neglectful than physically or sexually abusive. Those who have been previously abused or neglected themselves are more likely to be married and have children than those who were not (Tymchuk and Andron 1990). Children were not removed because of their parent's handicap per se. Nevertheless, a severe disability does lead to problems in parenting.

As yet, very little has been written about the links between learning disability and domestic violence. The literature that does exist focuses on disabled women (Mays 2006; Radford et al. 2006), or the effects of domestic violence on disabled children (Bentovim et al. 2009). Respond (the leading charity specialising in supporting victims and perpetrators of abuse with learning disabilities), together with Respect (an umbrella group for domestic violence perpetrator programmes in the UK), are currently piloting a group programme for learning-disabled adolescents who have used interpersonal violence in relationships. There remain many areas to be explored further, such as domestic violence in couples where both partners are learning disabled, or when children who are not learning disabled use violence against their learning-disabled parents.

The learning-disabled sexual offender

Bronya Booth and Maria Grogan (1990) in examining sexual offences by learning-disabled adults in the North West Region found that out of 76 sexual offenders, 73 were male and 3 female. The majority were in the 16–25 age-range and almost half were in the mild to moderate learning disability group. Only 15 per cent lived in hospital or prison and most lived in the parental home.

It is commonly agreed (Griffiths et al. 1985) that the nature of deviant sexual behaviour is similar for both learning-disabled and non-learning disabled offenders but the learning-disabled sex offender is less likely to reach the courts and therefore treatment (Breen and Turk 1991) and his or her crimes are more likely to be detected. However, there is some evidence that learning-disabled offenders can become more violent (Gilby et al. 1989) and are more likely to find male than female victims (Griffiths et al. 1985). There is also concern at the lack of attention paid to the emotional meaning and consequences of mild learning disability within the forensic system.

John (not his real name) was 22 when he was referred to Respond following the discovery of boy's underwear under his bed. John lived in a small residential care home for adults with learning disabilities and had grown up in care after having been removed from his parents, aged 7, following allegations that he and his 8-year-old brother had been sexually abused by them. John was referred for a forensic risk assessment in order to try and understand whether John was a risk to children. In the assessment sessions John talked about his phantasies of abducting a young boy and sexually assaulting him. He confided that he had had these types of phantasies since he was about 13 and that so far he had not acted upon his urges due to his fear of being locked up. He also admitted to having stolen the underwear at night from local gardens and said that he was very aware of where young boys that might become his victims lived. John also described how sad he was about not having seen his parents since he was removed and how lonely he was in his home and in his life in general. John was unable to conceive of his parents as having been anything other than benign and when asked about the abuse he said it 'hadn't been that bad'. John's case demonstrated a familiar pattern of unprocessed sexual trauma manifesting as dangerous sexualised behaviour. Fortunately for John he was referred for psychotherapeutic treatment and he was able to work through some of his trauma and to make the necessary links between this and his risky behaviours.

In working with a long-term psychoanalytic group of sex offenders with learning disabilities, Hollins and Sinason (2000) found they were re-enacting earlier experiences of being abused. Curen (2009) writes that many traumatised clients seen at Respond have internalised the idea of a protective shell in order to protect themselves from further abandonments like those experienced in childhood. Their previous experiences of separation and loss mean that issues of relating to others are mixed in with feelings of anxiety and of depression. In the case of sexual offenders a 'solution' to these internal conflicts is to employ sexualisation, which converts aggression to sadism (Campbell 1989; Glasser 1996). The intention to unconsciously destroy those people that have abandoned them is then converted into a wish to hurt and control that is acted out on their victims.

Signs and symptoms

All the usual range of signs and symptoms that apply to all children are relevant to this population. The lengthy list comprises almost every reason for referral of children to clinics: bedwetting, school phobia, stomach-ache, nightmares, deterioration in schoolwork, inability to concentrate, inappropriate sexualised behaviour, excessive masturbating, promiscuity, running away, drug addiction, prostitution, self-destructive behaviour, anorexia nervosa, abuse of younger children, etc. However, there is still an unwillingness to listen properly and believe what is being communicated.

Linda (not her real name), an 8-year-old severely learning-disabled girl, masturbated with a toothbrush every evening in her foster-home. She wet the bed each night and displayed a great deal of emotional disturbance after each access visit to her parents. The foster-mother was convinced that sexual abuse was taking place at the girl's home but no professional believed her. Indeed, one professional firmly stated, 'On no account should this child's hypersexual activity be seen as anything other than intrinsic to her brain damage'. Only when the child's desperate communications extended to her school classroom was a referral made to a child abuse team.

All too often such signs are dismissed because of a widespread belief among professionals that handicapped children masturbate solely to enjoy the physical relief it brings. Indeed, in some schools and centres, excessive public masturbation is treated solely with social skills or educational packages in the belief that the child lacks the knowledge of appropriate boundaries.

Many of the signs that apply to all children take on a different shape when applied to the learning-disabled child population. For example, it is widely understood that self-destructive behaviour is one of the possible sequelae of abuse. However, in the learning-disabled population, instead of alcohol or drugs to which there is less financial access, there can be self-mutilation, eye-poking, cutting of genitals and head-banging.

Access to psychotherapy

Any form of psychotherapy or counselling is still far too rare a resource both nationally and internationally for children and adults with a learning disability (Sinason 1991; 1992a; 1992b), but psychoanalytic psychotherapy is the rarest. When research was undertaken on self-injurious behaviour in children and adults with a learning disability in one region (Oliver et al. 1987) it was found that of 596 such children and adults only 12 were receiving any psychological help of which one was psychoanalytical.

It is adult survivors who face the greatest lack of resources: NHS child psychotherapy training schemes have gradually made space for children with a learning disability who have suffered abuse. However, although there has been a small increase in non-intensive work with such children, particularly those with autistic diagnoses, the number of intensive training cases is still relatively small.

Respond, together with the members of the Institute for the Psychotherapy of Disability (IPD), which was formed in 2000, wrote to all psychotherapy training organisations asking about their access for children and adults with severe learning disabilities and whether they were including them as training patients. To date there has hardly been any response. It is a commitment of the IPD to ensure inclusion and access in all psychotherapy trainings. Earlier this year the United Kingdom Council for Psychotherapy, the largest psychotherapy umbrella organisation, recognised Disability Psychotherapy as a speciality and hopefully this will lead to more patients with a disability being accepted as cases on psychotherapy training courses.

Until the last decade, very few psychoanalysts and psychoanalytic psychotherapists have either specialised in working with this client group or included them in their range of service users, let alone therapists from other backgrounds. The authors consider that, whether by implicit or explicit inclusion, the psychoanalytic history, like the political and educational history, points to a history of trauma. Lack of access to treatment, whether by unconscious exclusion or deliberate policy, whether consciously or unconsciously, malign or benevolent, in itself is a statement of untreatability.

Conclusion

However, change is happening, albeit slowly. An historic vote was taken at the Royal College of Psychiatry in May 2003, in which the need for access to treatment of psychotherapy was accepted and a major report on psychotherapy and learning disability was welcomed. The Council report (RCP 2004) demonstrated that people with learning disabilities can benefit from psychotherapy but that there was 'neither inclusion nor equity for this needy client group' (ibid.: 57). Anecdotally things have continued to change but the pace is very unhurried. The VVAPP programme properly included disability but many government department initiatives, e.g. the Cross-Government Action Plan on Sexual Violence and Abuse 2007 (HM Government 2007), pay little attention to the needs of people with learning disabilities, although as stated above they are often much more vulnerable and much less likely to be able to access appropriate services.

The government has a responsibility to make sure that the needs of this client group are given higher prominence in all relevant decision-making activities. The voluntary and statutory sectors are getting better at responding to the needs of this group but need better resources and champions in every part of the country who are passionate enough to drive change forward. The changes needed include professionals being better trained in order to provide appropriate psychological support and for families, carers and professionals to be better able to recognise abuse and to respond to it accordingly.

8.2 Physically disabled women

Jackie Barron and Nicola Harwin

Introduction

While all women and children are at risk from sexual and domestic violence, the nature and impact of such abuse on disabled women and children may be particularly severe. Not only do disabled women experience more abuse than non-disabled women throughout their lives from childhood onwards, but also disability and abuse interact and compound each other, increasing and widening the abuser's power and control, and at the same time making it much harder for the victims to seek help.

Disabled women, domestic and sexual violence: a summary of the issues

Research in this area has been somewhat limited, and disabled women have often been excluded from mainstream research (see Barile 2002). However, the studies available indicate that disabled women are at least twice as likely as non-disabled women to experience abuse, and some studies suggest a much greater prevalence of the experience of abuse among disabled women; for example, Sobsey (2000) cites a number of small-scale studies in the USA which suggest that women with developmental impairments experience sexual assault, in particular, between four and ten times more frequently than other women; see also Davis (2000). However, other studies have found that the prevalence of abuse was not much different between disabled and non-disabled women; see Nosek and colleagues (1997). Studies also suggest that the abuse is likely to be more severe and more prolonged, and that the kinds of abuse experienced are more diverse and wide-ranging, may be linked to the woman's impairments, and are more likely to involve humiliation, and sexual and financial abuse (Chenoweth, 1997; Depoy et al. 2003; Hague et al. 2008a, 2000b; Humphreys and Thiara 2002; James-Hanman 1998; Magowan 2003; Mays 2006; Nosek and Howland 1998; Nosek et al. 2001, 2006; Radford et al. 2005, 2006; Saxton et al. 2001). To quote from a report by the Australian organisation, Women with Disabilities Australia (WWDA):

A concise definition of violence in this area is made difficult by the pervasive nature of abuse against women with disabilities ... including unnecessary institutionalisation, denial of control over their bodies, lack of financial control, denial of social contact and community participation as well as physical, mental and sexual abuse.

(WWDA 2004: 4)

Abuse against disabled women may also be perpetrated by a wide range of potential abusers, including partners, former partners, other family members, personal assistants and carers (both paid and unpaid), acquaintances and – less frequently – strangers. It may take place in the woman's own home, in residential care or other institutional settings, or in a public place such as the street. Practices which, for example, force disabled women into sharing mixed-sex residential accommodation can both create vulnerability and dependence, and increase opportunities for abuse (see Radford et al. 2005; Roberto and Teaster 2005).

The first part of this chapter addresses domestic and sexual abuse against disabled women in their own homes, where the perpetrators are partners, former partners, other family members or personal assistants or other carers. Domestic violence includes physical, sexual, psychological or financial violence and abuse that takes place within an intimate or family-type relationship and that forms a pattern of coercive and controlling behaviour. It may include a range of abusive behaviours, not all of which are in themselves inherently 'violent' – for example, emotional abuse.

Most of the data for this chapter come from the recent Women's Aid study of physically disabled women and domestic violence, undertaken by researchers from the Universities of Bristol and Warwick (Hague et al. 2008a; 2008b). The research was undertaken between September 2005 and March 2008 by Professor Gill Hague and Dr Pauline Magowan from the Violence Against Women Research Group, University of Bristol and Dr Ravi Thiara from the Centre for the Study of Safety and Well-being at the University of Warwick. It was managed by Women's Aid and funded by the Big Lottery Fund. The aims of the research included developing further understandings of the needs of disabled women experiencing domestic violence, and investigating existing service provision (including identifying the gaps in such provision). Its focus was on the needs and experiences of women with physical and sensory impairments. The research was grounded in the social model of disability, in which disability is viewed as socially created. In this model – in contrast to the more pervasive medical model – the barriers experienced by disabled people are attributed to the failure (by organisations and other people) to take account of their needs. It is this failure that is truly disabling, not people's individual impairments. This model is also supported by the Department of Health, see for example, <http://www.dh.gov.uk/en/SocialCare/Deliveringadultsocialcare/Disability/index.htm>.

The research included an initial focus group and other consultation sessions with disabled women, interviews with key professionals and activists, two postal surveys with specialist providers (see below) and semi-structured interviews with disabled women who had experienced domestic and sexual abuse. The disabled women who were interviewed for this research had experienced a wide range of abuse, which had often continued over an extended period. The perpetrators included intimate partners, personal assistants (PAs), and family members, and some women had been abused by more than one person. (As others have also pointed out, paid personal assistants and other carers carry out a range of often very intimate tasks, qualifying them in effect to become part of the disabled women's 'family'; as such, they are also potential perpetrators of domestic abuse; see, for example, the website of the Public Health Agency of Canada: 'What makes women with disabilities particularly vulnerable to family violence?' <http://www.phac-aspc.gc.ca/ncfv-cnivf/publications/femdisab-eng.php>). All the respondents said that being disabled made the abuse worse, and also severely limited their capacity to escape or take other preventive measures.

The experiences of disabled women

The research emphasised that being disabled strongly affected the nature, extent and impact of abuse, and the pervasive nature of abuse perpetrated against disabled women was very apparent. Women's impairments were frequently used in the abuse: for example, mobility or communication devices may be removed, the victim may be deliberately isolated, and vital aspects of care may be undertaken abusively, or not at all. Humiliation and belittling are often an integral part of the abuse, and were found to be particularly prevalent.

> Oh yes, he would drag me along the floor because I couldn't walk or get away that was how it would start, the way it always went. He'd insult me with all those names, 'you spassy' and so on, 'who'd want to marry you?' And he smashed me against the wall, shouting insults, you cripple, all that sort of thing.
>
> (This quote and the others in this chapter are from the disabled women interviewed for the above study.)

Current definitions of domestic violence may be too narrow to encompass the range of experiences of disabled women. Domestic violence typically involves a pattern of coercive and controlling behaviour, and when a woman is disabled, this can potentially increase the power differential between her and her abuser; see also Radford and colleagues (2005). Many abusers deliberately emphasised and reinforced the woman's dependence as a way of asserting and maintaining control.

>Because I can't feed myself and he would go out in the evenings deliberately and I wouldn't have eaten anything for a twenty-four hour period or more. So that wouldn't have happened to anybody that could feed themselves.

When the perpetrator was also the woman's carer, the abuse was particularly insidious and difficult to escape. Abuse from personal assistants and other carers (both paid and unpaid) was common. Disabled people are often treated as 'vulnerable' and incapable of making their own life choices, and the perpetrator can build on this in order to persuade the disabled woman she would be unable to live without him, and/or that she is unlikely to find anyone else to care for her as he does.

>Well, people are going to use whatever they can to abuse you, so whatever they can. If you've got mobility problems, that's a good one! Ideal for an abuser ——, isn't it, you can't get away or fight back, perfect.

It seems that some men deliberately target disabled women – seeing them as particularly easy to control, and perhaps as a potential source of income, also.

>I think some see us [disabled women] as sort of children and all, think we're women that need looking after a bit more. And those are the men that are more likely to become controlling and take it too far you know … we're very cautious about men and their motives and why they want to be with us.

Financial abuse was particularly common with carers often taking women's personal allowances, benefits and other money: 'I wasn't allowed any food for the children. I had to take that from child allowance'.

Disabled women faced particular barriers in obtaining help. Service provision was often inaccessible, inappropriate or unavailable. Additional factors included isolation (which is often deliberately created), and the responses from agencies which was often one of disbelief that disabled women could experience abuse – particularly notable in cases of sexual abuse. Professionals to whom women reported the abuse often did not take them seriously, or made them feel guilty.

>People pity him because he is taking care of you and so noble. So people are reluctant to criticise this saint or to think he could be doing these terrible things. And possibly as well as that there's a sort of I think an idea … people don't really 'see' disabled women. And people don't easily see a disabled woman as a wife, partner, and mother. So I think for some people it's hard to think well this might be a woman who's being sexually or physically abused by her partner, … because disabled women don't have sex, do they?

There were additional problems if women needed to leave home to escape their abuser. Care packages were not easily transferable to different areas, or their homes might have been adapted for them, and women feared losing their independence if they moved away. They also had a particular fear that their children might be taken away, as they might be seen to be unable to look after them alone.

In addition, many disabled women have been encouraged from childhood to be passive and compliant – particularly so if they have spent time in an institutional setting. All this means that they are less likely to report the abuse to anyone; and if they do report it – for example, to the police, social services or healthcare professionals – their reports are more likely to be ignored rather than acted on.

The response from service providers

One of the issues explored within the Women's Aid research was the extent, nature and availability of service provision offering support, information and accommodation to disabled women experiencing domestic violence. To this end, a postal survey was undertaken of all domestic and sexual violence organisations within England (342 in total) and all organisations of and for disabled people, both locally and nationally (322 organisations in all at that time).

Seven per cent of women using domestic violence services were noted as having physical and sensory impairments.[1] Thirty-eight per cent of specialist domestic violence organisations offered some form of specific services to disabled women. These were primarily 'structural' though some refuges were able to offer specialised emotional support. Only three projects had disabled staff in post. Organisations were most likely to interpret disability access solely in terms of wheelchair access – which they often found difficult to achieve within existing resources and due to the nature of the accommodation they were using – and tended to overlook the equally important need to be accessible to women with sensory impairments.

It was apparent that – while appropriate service provision has improved in recent years – it is often patchy and sometimes minimal, and a significant proportion admitted that, at the time of the survey,[2] they were not yet fully compliant with the Disability Discrimination Act 2005.

At the time of this survey, there were still many domestic violence organisations which had hardly addressed the issue at all and, overall, knowledge and awareness of the needs of disabled women need substantial development. The researchers emphasised that the needs of disabled women must be embedded at both operational and management levels as a core issue in domestic violence services, in order to build on the good work already undertaken in some projects.

The response of disability organisations was even more uneven. Very few organisations for disabled people considered that it was part of their remit to deal with domestic violence at all, and their limited resources certainly made it difficult for them to address the issue. Less than a quarter of those responding[3] had specific provision for disabled women experiencing abuse, and only four organisations employed dedicated staff with domestic violence expertise. The vast majority said they were rarely approached for support for this issue but that if this occurred, they would automatically signpost to specialist agencies; and while this might certainly be the best response in many cases, it relied on the availability of appropriate specialist services, and the ability of the client to access them quickly and safely. The few disability organisations that were providing information and support to disabled women experiencing domestic and sexual violence were clear that other such organisations also needed to develop an improved awareness of the issues, in particular by building links with local and national specialist services in order to improve their future response. They concluded that disabled people's organisations should take on the issue of domestic violence as both a management and an operational concern.

How should health and social care professionals respond to disabled women experiencing abuse?

The specialist domestic violence and disability organisations included in this research all operate within the voluntary non-profit sector. However, the statutory sector also has a large part to play in responding to the needs of abused disabled women – and the health, mental health and social care services clearly have a particular role here.

Many disabled women have experienced a lifetime of abuse, hence they may not clearly identify it as such, and this acknowledgement to themselves is a precondition of reporting it to others. If the perpetrator continually justifies his behaviour, denies that it is abusive, or tells the woman it is her own fault, keeping silent and putting up with it is the almost inevitable outcome.

The relative isolation of disabled people, often reinforced by their abusers, means that their contacts with health and social care professionals are often crucial. Disclosing abuse is made even harder for disabled women when the professionals from whom they might expect support and help do not make it easy, or indeed possible, to disclose what is being done to them.

Health and social care professionals may not realise that domestic violence is a major issue for disabled women, and therefore they rarely, if ever, take time to ask them about it. They may also consistently fail to provide an opportunity to see the woman alone without her carer, making disclosure difficult or, when the carer is the perpetrator, impossible and/or potentially dangerous. They may assume, or it may be implied by the perpetrator, that any injuries they notice are the results of the disability, as in cases where the woman may bruise or break bones easily, or if the abuser claims she fell while getting out of her wheelchair. If the abuser is himself disabled, they may assume that he cannot be a serious threat: or they may inhibit disclosure because they are unsure how to respond, or are under pressure to get things done quickly. Jacki Pritchard (2000) in looking at the abuse of older women identified many of the same issues, which apply to all disabled women, regardless of their age. In addition, well-meaning professionals may 'take charge' and, in responding to the disabled woman as a 'vulnerable person', make decisions on her behalf, without properly consulting her, thus compounding the disempowerment already imposed by the perpetrator of the abuse; see Mullender (1996: 134).

For these and other reasons, women may distrust the responses of health and social care professionals and will therefore be reluctant to disclose that they are being abused. In particular, they fear they may lose their independence, or that their children might be taken away, a fear that in some cases, at least, may be justified. For example, one woman in the Women's Aid study was able to have her children back with her only because she had a partner, albeit an abusive one. Another woman had only narrowly managed to prevent her daughter being taken into foster care. Other women, who had to leave home because of danger to their lives, had left their children behind (sometimes with a violent father) because they did not know whether the accommodation they were going to would be able to house their children as well as themselves. In one such case, social services and other agencies said nothing could be done and refused to help in getting the child back, and the woman concerned was sure the response would have been different if she had not been disabled.

Conclusion

Disabled women facing abuse experience a *greater need* for services, accompanied by far *less provision*, so lose out on both counts. For too long, their needs have been ignored, and a cultural change is now well overdue.

The Women's Aid study and others undertaken both in the UK and internationally have clearly demonstrated that the needs of disabled women are often neglected by service providers, policy-makers and funders. This situation needs to be addressed urgently. One approach is to embed the needs of abused disabled women and children at both operational and management levels in all organisations, and in particular within those in the specialist disability and domestic violence sectors.

However, the development of such practice often depends on the wider strategic and partnership agenda, both nationally and in the relevant local areas. In particular, the removal of the ring-fence around Supporting People funding and the introduction of competitive tendering for specialist domestic violence services is likely to slow down the introduction of initiatives aimed at improving service provision for disabled women and children within this sector. Priorities for local funding and decisions on allocation are now determined by local area agreements (LAAs). Depending on the local situation, the needs of disabled women experiencing domestic abuse might potentially be highlighted within these agreements, if the key agencies within the statutory and the voluntary sector were able to agree on the issues. However, current indicators relating to domestic violence are criminal justice-focused, and do not specifically include the provision of local women's domestic violence organisations so there is much less scope to incorporate wider aspects of support – including disability issues.

Recommendations

- The development of more comprehensive service provision in all sectors for disabled women experiencing domestic and sexual violence;
- Effective awareness-raising in all sectors about the impact of domestic and sexual abuse on disabled women and children;
- Mandatory training for all health and social care professionals and those working in disability organisations and in the domestic violence sector on how to respond appropriately to disabled women and children who have experienced domestic and sexual violence and abuse;
- The involvement of disabled women in all service development in these areas;
- The development of more effective partnership working among domestic violence organisations, disability organisations and statutory sector health and social care services;
- The integration of appropriate quality standards for specialist domestic and sexual violence services within commissioning and procurement frameworks.

Notes

1 These statistics were collected in a day count of women using domestic violence services on one day in 2006. More recent figures will shortly become available from a similar day count undertaken in 2009.
2 The postal survey was undertaken in 2006 – very soon after the implementation of the Act – and it is very likely that most services are now fully compliant with the legislation.
3 The response rate for disability organisations was particularly low, perhaps indicating the limited importance they gave to the issue. Many who did respond said simply that they do no work on this issue.

8.3 Disabled children

Ruth Marchant

This part of Chapter 8 explores the health and mental health effects of the abuse of disabled children, by presenting the stories of three different children and young people and reflecting on the impact of childhood impairment and disabling barriers on their experiences. The three stories untangle some of the risk factors for disabled children, explore the strong association between childhood maltreatment and childhood impairment and consider the additional barriers faced by disabled children in getting help and accessing support. The conclusion summarises the legislation and guidance that provides the current framework for safeguarding disabled children in the UK and giving practical pointers for best practice in tackling the health and mental health effects of the abuse of disabled children.

The following principles underpin the chapter:

- Disabled children have the same fundamental rights and basic needs as all children, but have additional vulnerabilities in terms of both the risk of abuse and the health and mental health effects of abuse. Most of these vulnerabilities are created rather than an inevitable result of the child's impairments.
- Many disabled children also have additional needs, in relation to safeguarding and communication.
- Getting things right for disabled children will improve practice with all children and families, by creating more inclusive and more competent services.

Defining childhood disability

There is wide variation in the way childhood disability is defined and recorded in England, therefore the incidence or prevalence of childhood disability cannot be estimated with any confidence (Mooney et al. 2008: Read et al. 2008). Defining and recording childhood disability has proven very problematic.

The Children Act 1989 required local authorities to identify the extent to which there are children in need within their area and to maintain a register of disabled children within their area (the Children Act 1989 sch 2 para 1(1) and para 2(1)). Attempts to create registers of disabled children have hit serious implementation issues, partly because of confusion about definitions, and partly because parents feared the association with child protection registers.

Children's chances of being defined as disabled vary widely according to where they live: there is no consensus on what should be included in local definitions of disability. For example, a child in England with an autistic spectrum disorder has an 88 per cent chance of being defined as disabled, but this reduces to 55 per cent with dyspraxia and 53 per cent with Attention Deficit Hyperactivity Disorder (ADHD) (Read et al. 2008).

Disability and abuse

The lack of clarity and consistency about definitions of disability creates a confusing context, but nevertheless there is clearly a strong association between childhood maltreatment and childhood impairment:

- Disabled children are more likely to be abused.
- Abused children are more likely to become disabled.
- The abuse of disabled children is less likely to be picked up.
- Abused disabled children face additional barriers in accessing services and support.

A retrospective US study of 50,000 children found an unequivocal link between childhood maltreatment and disability, with disabled children being 3.4 times more likely to be abused: a 31 per cent prevalence rate against 9 per cent for non-disabled children (Sullivan & Knutson 2000). Smaller-scale studies in the US have also reported significant levels of abuse of deaf children (Sullivan et al. 1987) and children with Autism and Asperger's Syndrome (Mandell et al. 2005).

Research in the UK has been limited but a number of studies have indicated similar levels of abuse and neglect to that found in the US. Higher levels of maltreatment of disabled young people than of their non-disabled peers were found in a study of 3000 young people aged 18–24 (Cawson 2002), for example, 22 per cent of disabled young people reported experiencing sexual abuse compared to 15 per cent of the sample as a whole.

There is a widespread lack of local and national data on disabled children who are subject to safeguarding children procedures. Cooke and Standen (2002) surveyed local authorities across the UK and found that only a third of authorities had specific guidelines for safeguarding disabled children and only 50 per cent recorded whether an abused child had a disability. Despite 50 per cent of authorities reportedly collecting these data only 10 were able to provide figures on the number of reported cases of abuse of disabled children. Practice was very variable.

There are also very limited data regarding the characteristics of children who have been the subject of serious case reviews. Brandon and colleagues (2009) found 14 children (8 per cent) of their full sample of 189 children who had been subject to a serious case review were disabled prior to the incident leading to the serious case review. This figure is a slight increase in the figure of 8 children (5 per cent) in the previous study of 161 children (Brandon et al. 2008).

Figures from the 2005 Children in Need Census (DES 2006a) illustrate that disabled children are over-represented among the looked-after population, making up 10 per cent of all children in care, and only around 5 per cent of the overall population. Disabled children are also more likely than non-disabled children to be looked after because of abuse or neglect.

In summary, disabled children are particularly vulnerable to abuse, yet are seriously under-represented in child protection systems. This paradox in itself contributes to their increased vulnerability, which is explored further through the three stories below.

Early pick up: Nat's story

Nat lived with her mother; her parents separated very early in her life. Nat had no contact with her father. Nat's mother struggled financially, and was treated several times for depression. There was professional concern early in Nat's life, initially about her growth (she was below the 10th percentile on weight and height) and later about her development (she was very late to sit, walk and talk). At the age of two Nat was diagnosed with autism and severe learning difficulties.

She was placed in the nursery class of a special school for children with a range of needs, and taxi transport was funded by the local authority. In addition, Nat was offered overnight breaks with a family carer once a month. Nat's mother made a new relationship with a man she met through a friend. He moved in with the family and began to provide financial support and help with Nat's care.

The pace of Nat's development improved significantly, particularly her language and her social skills. However, her behaviour became much more challenging, with violence towards herself, other children and adults: hitting, pinching and hair pulling. She also began to masturbate compulsively. These behaviours were seen variously as 'part and parcel' of her autism and learning difficulty, or a reaction to the many changes in her life. A basic behavioural management programme was put in place where the concerning behaviours were ignored and attention given to more positive behaviours.

When Nat was four, she had a urinary tract infection, and this led to the discovery that she had two different sexually transmitted diseases. All those involved in her day-to-day care – including school staff – were initially adamant that she could not be at risk of abuse, because her behaviour was so difficult and because she resisted having her pad changed with such violence that two adults were required.

Enquiries found that Nat's step-father had previous convictions for sexual assault and possession of pornographic images of children. It also emerged that concerns had been raised in the past about the behaviour of Nat's taxi driver, particularly his physical contact with young girls, although he had no convictions. The family providing overnight breaks had also recently accommodated a teenager with severe learning difficulties following concerns around sexual abuse in his own family, and he had spent time with Nat.

When presented with this information, Nat's mother's initial response was to deny that her partner could possibly present any risk. The local authority proposed an interim care order, but Nat's mother consented to her being placed with a foster-family on a voluntary basis. Nat was not felt to be able to give evidence and because the clinical findings were not specific it was not possible to press charges against any of those potentially involved.

Nat's behaviour became very disturbed. Her mother had contact with her twice a week, and with support from her family and social worker she decided to end the relationship with her partner and Nat was able to return home. Nat's behaviour became more settled, although she continued to injure herself and others, particularly men.

What can be learnt from Nat's story?

Nat's experiences can illustrate a great deal about how vulnerability is created. First, her story illustrates the links between poverty, social disadvantage, disability and abuse. These links are well established. There are more disabled children in groups already socially disadvantaged: Whatever system is used to classify disability, the number of disabled children in social class 5 households is twice that in social class 1 and there is a strong relationship between childhood disability and household income (Dobson and Middleton, 1998). Thus children affected by disability are at greater risk of living in poverty, with over half of families with disabled children living in or at the margins of poverty (Gordon et al. 2000). Families who are relatively financially secure are also more likely to descend into poverty when they have a disabled child (DRC 2006; EDCM 2007).

There is also a strong association between poverty and an increased risk of child maltreatment, particularly neglect and physical abuse (Dyson 2008).

Some of the most damaging experiences in the lives of disabled children, and their families, are not an inevitable consequence of the child's condition. Nat's story makes this very clear: her exposure to the risk of sexual abuse in several situations resulted from society's response to her needs, not directly from her impairments.

There are many reasons for disabled children becoming more vulnerable to abuse, including the higher number of adults involved in their lives; the greater time they spend away from their families; inadequate and poorly coordinated support services; isolation and a common failure to consult with and listen to disabled children about their experiences, and negative social attitudes towards disabled children – their lives and their experiences are commonly devalued and the strong emphasis on giving parents a break can reinforce this negative framing (Marchant and Jones 2008).

As the government has recently noted, it has 'traditionally' been the case that disabled children are likely to have poorer outcomes across a range of indicators compared to their non-disabled peers, including lower educational attainment, poorer access to health services and therefore poorer health outcomes, more difficult transitions to adulthood, and poorer employment outcomes (HM Treasury and DES 2007). Nat's story also makes clear how abuse can go unrecognised. Behaviours that would have raised serious concern in a non-disabled child – compulsive masturbation and extreme distress at intimate care – were responded to with a behaviour management programme.

Possible indicators of concern about children's safety or welfare can thus be denied, ignored, attributed to a child's impairment or condition or even somehow seen as evidence that a child could not be abused.

Finally, Nat's story demonstrates the barriers within the criminal justice system, where young children's evidence is often unheard or discredited, particularly if they also have a communication impairment.

Investigation: Marjit's story

Marjit was a nine-year-old boy living with his family. He had a learning disability and also a significant speech impairment resulting from a cleft palate. Marjit attended a mainstream primary school where he had additional help in class.

His older brother, Tuyen, had been an important ally and support for Marjit at school, particularly at breaktimes and walking to and from school. As Tuyen moved up to secondary school Marjit's mother wanted to walk with him, but he said he would be teased by the other children and insisted on walking alone.

Marjit sometimes arrived back from school very hungry, and sometimes with bruises or damaged clothing. He said that some older boys had taken his lunch money and chased him, but begged his parents not to contact the school.

A few weeks later Marjit arrived home badly hurt, with severe bruising to his face, two broken ribs and cuts to his hands. He said he had been beaten up by older boys in the alleyway near to school, and they had called him 'a spasser' and 'a stupid paki'.

Marjit's parents called the school and then the police. The incident was investigated and because of Marjit's age and additional needs, he was interviewed by trained officers with the help of an intermediary. The interview was recorded. Despite his distress and his communication difficulties, Marjit gave a clear account of what had happened and a detailed description of the older boys.

The police, with the help of the school, were able to identify the boys and interviewed them. The boys were also given fixed-term exclusions from school. The file of the investigation was presented to the Crown Prosecution Service, who decided charges could not be brought because Marjit was unlikely to withstand cross-examination.

The older boys returned to school and Marjit became increasingly withdrawn and anxious. He was escorted to and from the school door each day by his parents and he went to an indoor club at breaktimes. Marjit lost weight and had difficulty sleeping. His school work suffered and he became despairing and despondent.

What can be learnt from Marjit's story?

Marjit's experiences demonstrate the double jeopardy of racism and disablism: disabled children report a much higher incidence of bullying (Mencap 2007) and children from minority ethnic groups are vulnerable to specific kinds of bullying (DES 2006b) Marjit's story makes clear the challenge that is represented by the creation of diverse communities that are safe for all.

Disabled children and those with visible medical conditions can be twice as likely as their peers to become targets for bullying behaviour (Office of the Children's Commissioner 2006).Two out of five children on the autistic spectrum report being bullied at school (National Autistic Society 2006). An even higher proportion of people with a learning disability experience some form of bullying, with over two-thirds experiencing it on a regular basis (Mencap 2007). Government guidance on Bullying involving Children with Special Educational Needs and Disabilities (DCSF 2008a) notes that disabled children may be more at risk of bullying because of their impairment (for example, they may be less able to move away or they may have cognitive impairments which make anticipation and avoidance difficult).

Marjit's story also makes clear the cumulative impact of 'low level' abuse in terms of damaging a child's sense of self and thus increasing a child's vulnerability in different settings. The experience of being bullied can affect a young person's social relationships and have a corrosive and damaging impact on their self-esteem, mental health, social skills and progress at school (Murray and Osborne 2009). Some children learn to expect bad treatment, which places them at additional risk in the long term. The lack of self-esteem resulting from bullying can in itself make disabled children more vulnerable to abuse.

Marjit's story also demonstrates the depth of some of the barriers to justice: even with a careful police investigation, with special measures and a compelling account, the decision was made not to prosecute. This was a difficult decision for Marjit and his family to accept. Working Together (HM Government 2006) sets out the responsibilities of agencies to safeguard and promote the welfare of children. It has a specific section on the abuse of disabled children (Paragraphs 11.28–11.32) which highlights that disabled children may be especially vulnerable to abuse and guidance is also given on handling concerns about disabled children, and communicating with disabled children. The government has also issued additional practice guidance on safeguarding disabled children (Murray and Osborne 2009).

This guidance enabled Marjit's account to be heard, and the special measures for vulnerable and intimidated witnesses introduced by The Youth Justice and Criminal Evidence Act 1999 (http://www.opsi.gov.uk/Acts/acts1999/ukpga_19990023_en_1) were also relevant for Marjit, who would have been eligible for special measures on two separate grounds. The Act defines vulnerable witnesses as all child witnesses under 17 years and any witness whose quality of evidence is likely to be diminished because they suffer from a mental disorder; have a significant impairment of intelligence and social functioning (e.g. a learning disability); or have a physical disability or are suffering from a physical disorder.

From April 2008 the last special measure – the use of an intermediary – was rolled out nationally and this is addressing some of the barriers that have existed for disabled children in the court setting.

Finally, Marjit's story reflects the barriers within support structures and services, which can make it more difficult for disabled young people to access appropriate support, particularly with their emotional and mental health needs.

Getting the right help: Ollie's story

Ollie was 14 and had a significant hearing impairment and mild cerebral palsy. He could walk unaided, but physical tasks were very difficult for him. Ollie had some limited speech but communicated mostly through sign, using a mix of British Sign Language (BSL) and sign-supported English (SSE).

Ollie was the oldest of four children. Throughout his early years, Ollie was bullied and belittled by his father, who blamed Ollie's mother for what he called their 'defective' son. His parents had disagreed about whether Ollie should attend an aural school to learn to access spoken language, or a signing school, and he changed primary schools several times.

Ollie's mother was subject to many violent attacks from Ollie's father, and when Ollie was 12 she left the family home and moved into a refuge with the children. The staff at the refuge offered skilled support to Ollie's siblings, but they were unable to communicate in sign. The family were rehoused to a new area and the children were placed at new schools. Ollie was placed at a mainstream secondary school with support.

Ollie's mother and staff at his school became concerned about his increasing isolation, his extreme mood swings and about some aspects of his behaviour. Ollie often withdrew completely, spending many hours alone in his room, refusing to eat, to respond to others or to attend school. He also began to cut his arms and legs with a razor blade.

Ollie initially refused therapy, until he was introduced to a therapist who was Deaf and a native BSL user. He then engaged enthusiastically and over time built a strong relationship in which he could explore some of his feelings and experiences. Ollie explained through sign and drawings that he felt responsible for his family's problems. He saw his cerebral palsy as a punishment for wrongdoing, and his deafness as something 'bad' and a source of great shame to him and his family. He told the therapist that he thought often about suicide and death.

A few months later Ollie's father made a contact order application through the courts, seeking contact with the three younger children but not with Ollie. With his therapist's help Ollie wrote a long letter to his father about all that had happened and how he felt. He then chose to burn the letter. Soon after this Ollie sought contact with Deaf young people and built new friendships at school and at a Deaf club.

What can Ollie's story teach us about the effects of domestic violence and abuse on disabled children?

Domestic violence can have a devastating impact on children, even if they are not subject to physical violence themselves (Mullender et al. 2002).

The intersection of disability and vulnerability is also made clear in Ollie's story. His father's perception of Ollie's impairments was part of what made him vulnerable and his struggle with his own identity reflects this understanding. Achieving a positive sense of identity as a Deaf or disabled young person presents particular challenges (Cross, 1999; Marchant

2008; Marchant and Jones 1999) and relationships with Deaf or disabled adults can be crucially important.

Ollie's story also demonstrates how Deaf or disabled children may be particularly vulnerable to the effects of abuse and how existing services may be inaccessible to these children. Increasing the accessibility of services requires a range of interventions in terms of attitudes and competence as well as physical resources and buildings.

Pointers to better practice

Enough is known to do things differently. Disabled children have the same fundamental rights and basic needs as all children. The same principles, the same guidance and the same laws apply. There is no need to begin from a different place.

It is crucial to remember that some of the most damaging aspects of the lives of disabled children are not an inevitable consequence of the child's condition or impairments. The five outcomes in Every Child Matters (be healthy; stay safe; enjoy and achieve; make a positive contribution; achieve economic well-being) are relevant for all children, but are much harder to achieve for some children than others. Disabled children have the same 'ordinary' wishes and needs as other children (i.e., to live at home with their families, go to school, spend time with their friends, and participate in leisure and community activities with family and peers) but they face major barriers on all levels, so that getting these 'ordinary' things remains extraordinarily difficult (Marchant et al. 2007).

- Plan inclusively – so disabled children are part of every local and national initiative, and added on afterwards;
- Involve disabled children and young people in planning;
- Assess in context – crucially addressing the child and family's wider situation as well as the child's individual needs, and consider the interaction between all of these;
- Assess carefully – the more complex the child's needs or situation, the more competent and robust the assessment process should be;
- Be clear about values – the absence of explicit values can lead to a dangerous tolerance of poor care and damaging experiences. As Read and colleagues note: 'in almost all aspects of their lives, experiences that would be regarded as too narrow, unsettling, exclusionary or damaging for a non-disabled child have often not even seemed to require justification for their disabled peers' (Read et al. 2006: 33).

Patterns of care that would generally cause serious concern are not unusual for disabled children. For example, Jason at the age of seven sleeps in four different places every month: residential school; home; link family and respite care unit. He also has frequent hospital admissions. With most seven-year-olds, such a fragmented pattern of care would cause serious concern. Similarly, in an average week, Jodie has more than 25 adults involved in her everyday support and care: her mum and dad; three home care workers; two community nurses; a taxi driver and escort; a teacher and three classroom assistants; two lunchtime helpers; a physiotherapist and assistant; and a team of eight day and night staff at a residential respite care unit. There are another 16 professionals involved on an occasional basis. Again, such discontinuity would cause very serious concern for most children, but is often accepted without question for disabled children (Marchant 2009).

Responding to the needs of disabled children can have a positive impact on safeguarding services at many levels: getting things right for children with more complex needs will improve practice with all children.

9 Abuse by professionals

Sarah Barter-Godfrey

Introduction

This chapter considers abuse by professionals, that is, perpetrators who are not friends or family nor strangers, but people that act in a professional capacity and through that profession come into contact with their victims. Abuse by professionals can range in type and pathology equivalent to any other group of offenders. However, as representatives of a profession, the effects of broken trust and betrayal can be amplified to include the whole of that profession, for failing to prevent the abuse and frequently for failing to respond appropriately to allegations. Abuse by professionals harms the social fabric and the uneven distribution of power allocated to professions, in particular their capacity to cover up misconduct, and can lead to a severe undoing of the social contract.

The term 'abuse' is used here with wide interpretation, to include exploitation, coercion and harassment, as well as violence and neglect. Various definitions are relevant and in particular the following excerpts are useful for understanding how abuse is currently conceptualised in research and commentary:

> Also called 'sexual coercion' sexual exploitation is best defined in the context of a violation of professional ethics. It occurs when a person in power takes advantage of the dependence and vulnerability of a 'client' who is placed in or voluntarily adopts a position where personal control and power are limited in order that the 'client' may benefit from the expertise of the person in power. It is always the responsibility of the person in power to avoid sexual behavior in these relationships because: (a) it is a violation of role expectations; (b) it is a misuse of authority and power; (c) it takes advantage of vulnerability and dependence; and (d) meaningful consent is impossible, since consent to sexual activity can only occur in an atmosphere of mutuality and equality.
>
> (Chibnall et al. 1998: 144)

> Sexual harassment is often defined as any sexually related behavior that is unwelcome, offensive, or that fails to respect the rights of others.
>
> (McDuff 2008: 298)

> '[S]exual exploitation' is defined as 'any actual or attempted abuse of a position of vulnerability, differential power, or trust, for sexual purposes, including, but not limited to, profiting monetarily, socially or politically from the sexual exploitation of another'. 'Sexual abuse' is defined as 'actual or threatened physical intrusion of a sexual nature, whether by force or under unequal or coercive conditions'.
>
> (UN 2005: 7–8)

Abuse by professionals includes the use of power and position to access victims, enable abuse, exacerbate vulnerability, inhibit disclosure and evade consequence for the perpetrator. Individual perpetration is dependent on the individual's role and the context within which that role is constructed and understood. As Marcotte states: 'individual agency depends on the integrity of the social institution' (Marcotte 2008: 36). Therefore in this chapter abuse by professionals is considered to be multi-faceted, along the dimensions of: people who use their professional standing to facilitate abuse; professions that use their institutional standing to conceal (and thereby facilitate) abuse; and professional practice that fails to prevent or redress abuse.

Abuse is widespread across society, and the dimensions for enabling abuse have the potential to be applied to almost any institution or organisation, and it is hoped to draw out general principles on the emergence and prevention of abuse by professionals. It is not possible in the scope of a single chapter to adequately represent all professions that may have abusers within their ranks or that fail to prevent abuses within their practices. Instead, this chapter looks at four professional groups that have notably high rates of recognised abuse and that make a unique contribution to our understanding of abuse by professionals. These are: religious institutions, armed forces, health and therapeutic professionals, and prison and corrections officers. These will be considered in turn and then finally principles of abuse-promoting and abuse-preventing features of institutions and professions will be drawn together.

Religious institutions

The chapter begins by looking at abuse by professionals within religious institutions, partly because of the high-profile scandals of the last two decades from the US, Australia and Ireland, but also because of the emerging evidence of multi-directional harassment and abuse-promoting conduct within faith-based communities.

Across the 1990s and 2000s, widespread allegations of child abuse perpetrated by Catholic priests, predominantly in the US, and institutionalised abuse in Catholic reformatory schools in Ireland came to light (Commission to Inquire into Child Abuse 2009; USCCB 2004). There are strong parallels between the two sets of abuses: sexual and physical abuses were perpetrated by clergy and church staff, children were intimidated and found it difficult to disclose their abuses, and allegations were rarely reported to police. Religious authorities would relocate clergy rather than remove them from service when abuses were known to occur, there was reluctance from religious authorities to acknowledge a systematic problem or intervene in individual cases of known abuse, and deference to religious institutions permitted the proliferation of abuses (ibid.).

'Clericalism', the belief that clergy are 'essentially different from the laity and ... men set apart by God' (Doyle 2006: 190) has been argued to be abuse-promoting in religious communities. First, androcentrism and patriarchy, vital to the structure and spread of abuse perpetrated by clergy, established clergy as authority figures who could not be disobeyed, in a belief system where obedience is a virtue and sex is a sin (Doyle 2006; Sands 2003). Secondly, a priest was able to use his clerical status as part of the grooming of a victim, placing him under 'religious duress' to submit to abuses. His victim would take on self-blame for enabling a priest to sin, and was rarely empowered to disclose the abuse for fear of punishment or disbelief (Doyle 2006). Thirdly, 'the hierarchical leadership knew, covered up, and even facilitated sexual abuse by moving known perpetrators from parish to parish and diocese to diocese' (Doyle 2006: 191), and disclosed offences 'were managed with a view to minimising the risk of public disclosure and consequent damage to the institution' (Commission to Inquire into Child Abuse 2009: executive summary), so that institutional responses to abuse were in favour of the offender and the institution, and not victim-centred. Additionally, lay authorities were deferential and lenient (Doyle 2006; Commission to Inquire into Child Abuse 2009), at least in part because of the acceptance of clergy and religious institutions as socially and morally superior, with institutional interests that outweighed the threat to the safety and well-being of individual children.

While clericalism is a persuasive explanation for the pervasiveness of abuse within religious institutions that was colluded with by authorities who failed to respond appropriately to allegations and evidence of abuse, it is important not to ignore the responsibility of the individual perpetrators. The John Jay study was paid for and endorsed by the United States Conference of Catholic Bishops, and sought to examine 'the nature and scope of the problem of sexual abuse of minors by clergy' (USCCB 2004: np), on the basis of information in alleged offenders' files. Victims had an average age of 12.6 years, 85 per cent of victims were aged 11–17 years, 50 per cent were aged 11–14 years and 80 per cent of the victims were boys (Cartor et al. 2008; Marcotte 2008; USCCB 2004). On-file allegations implicated between 3 per cent and 6 per cent of priests across the US, with little variation by region; of those who had allegations on file, 6 per cent have had police investigations and 2 per cent had served prison sentences at the time of reporting in 2004 (USCCB 2004). Comparing priests who abused children younger than 11 years old and those who abused children aged 12–17 years indicated some difference in offending patterns, with differences in place of initial contact, place of offending and specific offending behaviours (Cartor et al. 2008). Additionally it was suggested that a minority of priests did not discriminate by age, offending in both pre- and peri-pubescent age groups, and that this group were more heterogeneous in their offending patterns.

With one in five of victims identified in the John Jay data aged 10 years or younger at the time of abuse, it has been argued that in general priest offenders are not paedophiles per se, but hebephiles or ephebrophiles (attracted to pubescent minors or adolescents) (Cartor et al. 2008). When compared to non-clergy sex offenders, clergy offenders appear to abuse older victims, as well as a far greater proportion of victims being male, and tend to be older and better educated than 'typical' sex offenders (Langevin et al. 2000). Further, when clergy and non-clergy offenders are matched by demographic and educational factors, clergy offenders tend to use more force and fewer public instances (for example, outdoors or group sexual activities) than non-clergy offenders. The presence of greater force is also associated with delayed disclosure of abuse by the victim, and overall, clergy offenders tend to have later or an absence of criminal charges compared to 'typical' sex offenders (Langevin et al. 2000). Given the differences in victim characteristics, offending patterns, offender characteristics and the social positioning of clergy, it may be that clinical understanding of child abuse and appropriate interventions needs to be specialised in order to respond effectively to abuses perpetrated by clergy and religious institutions.

It is not only minors that are abused within religious institutions. Male and female clergy in protestant churches report sexual harassment, with female clergy experiencing greater harassment and in particular, younger, single and those serving in more conservative congregations, experiencing greatest sexual harassment (McDuff 2008). In various American surveys, over 70 per cent of Methodist clergywomen and female Rabbis have reported sexual harassment (Chibnall et al. 1998). It has been proposed that younger and more career-oriented women, particularly in job roles where women have only been recently introduced, are perceived to be a threat to male dominance or authority and as such are vulnerable to harassment as a reaction to the 'threat' that they present (De Coster et al. 1999; McDuff 2008). This may go some way to explaining the comparatively higher levels of abuse of female clergy (and also, as discussed in the next section, the abuse of women in the armed forces). However, sexual harassment has also been documented within traditional and long-established female religious roles, with 12 per cent of nuns reporting sexual exploitation during their religious life (Chibnall et al. 1998). Prevalence of exploitation by priests was twice that of exploitation by nuns (6.2 per cent compared to 3.1 per cent), with one in ten nuns reporting unwanted sexual attention from another nun during religious life. The outcomes for the victim appeared to be different depending on whether the sexual harassment was seen to be hetero- or homosexual: 'psychological consequences declined significantly when the exploitation was heterosexual, but remained uniformly elevated when the exploitation was of a homosexual nature' (ibid.: 154). This is further indicative that clinical interventions and healing strategies for those abused within religious institutions need to be sensitive to religious teachings in order to understand the sequelae of abuse.

The clergy and religious institutions may also have a role in sustaining domestic abuse or intimate partner violence (IPV). Spirituality and faith can be a source of strength for women experiencing IPV, and women, particularly older women, may seek advice and guidance from their faith leaders during periods of domestic abuse (Beaulaurier et al. 2007; Copel 2008; Ware et al. 2003). However, several studies have identified that clergy responses are often unhelpful, ranging from avoidance through to victim-blaming and endorsement of the abusive partner. Clergy often encourage remaining within an abusive marriage, honouring the marriage and the husband, because marriage is first 'a promise with God and second with your partner' (Beaulaurier et al. 2007: 750), with specific advice to pray for the partner to change or to improve themselves and for the woman to better fulfil the subservient wife role in order to reduce abusive incidents (Copel 2008). As well as encouraging the woman to remain within the abusive marriage and take on a more fully submissive role (thus increasing her vulnerable position within the family), clergy often endorse 'interventions' that are perpetrator-centred rather than victim-centred, and in which the victim is expected to be an active participant, for example praying for the abuser (Ware et al. 2003). This approach is broadly contradicted by the findings of the Delphi consultation within VVAPP discussed in Part II, which endorses victim-centred approaches that prioritise the victim's safety and healing within their own lives, and places the perpetrator as responsible for their own behaviour and behavioural change.

This emphasis on marriage as a religious duty and a sacred commitment is not unique to a specific faith and the major world religions share a tendency towards male leadership, with women positioned as less close to god, through exclusion from rituals and leadership roles, and positioned as subservient or inferior to her husband in a marriage (Levitt and Ware 2006). A study that sought responses from religious leaders from Christianity, Judaism and Islam in the US identified that inappropriate responses from religious leaders can sustain abusive relationships, both through discouraging the victim from leaving and by substantiating abusive beliefs about the subservience of women and the importance of 'wifely submission' (ibid.: 1178). Some of the religious leaders in the sample found the teaching of (female) submission problematic, whereas others felt that it was not problematic when it was taught alongside righteous or compassionate (male) leadership; again this latter interpretation places the power for choosing to stop or resist IPV with the victim rather than the perpetrator. A similar approach is often used by pastoral or biblical counsellors, when women experiencing IPV seek help and counselling from Christian counsellors. Pastoral counselling places the emphasis on the victim to 'grow', and in particular spiritually grow, out of their distress, and victims are often expected to forgive their abusers and seek forgiveness for their own sins to heal their distress (Fouque and Glachan 2000). Biblical counselling is 'authoritative and prescriptive ... directive and disciplining' (ibid.: 202), and for people who have experienced both mainstream and Christian counselling, biblical counsellors are perceived to be more directive and exert greater power, were trusted less and in particular those who work in pairs were rated more negatively. People in 'deliverance' ministries, i.e. those that work to deliver someone from their inner demons, especially felt that they were to blame for their distress. Again, these approaches are contradicted by the VVAPP findings, which suggest effective and safe healing after abuse comes from victim-centred approaches that do not place blame on the victim, and instead offer the victim choices about how to heal and seek to re-empower in non-directive ways.

In this section it has become clear that, within religious institutions, leaders and followers are both at risk of harassment, and children have been at particular risk of being abused. Clericalism and teaching of subservience have been identified as possible abuse-promoting features of religious institutions, and many parts of religious life have been demonstrated to be poorly equipped to prevent abuse or provide appropriate pathways to healing once abuse has occurred. However, the importance of faith and access to religious life and connection to god should not be underestimated and victims' spiritual needs should be taken into account within abuse-prevention and remediation strategies.

Military institutions

That violence is associated with the armed forces is perhaps a little unsurprising – armies are bodies of legitimised violence, honed aggression and expedient application of threat or actual harm for the protection of peace and nation. However, it is also clear that this aggression 'spills over' onto non-legitimate and non-military targets, with members of the armed forces abusing 'their own' or abusing their positions when occupying a front line. For young members of the armed forces, the military may take on the role of family, and indeed their training may encourage this; bullying in this scenario may therefore be akin to forms of domestic violence. Physical and sexual assault are used in military settings as part of the initiation of new recruits. In the Russian army 'dedovschchina', the institutional practice of abuse and harassment of young new recruits with regular violence, rape and assault, has been associated with suicide and desertion (Herspring 2005). In other countries, enforced heterosexuality within the military percolates through to the expression of a 'brutal masculinity' (Kelly 2000: 47) and there have been various scandals of routine sexual harassment, bullying in military training colleges, and suspicious suicides of young officers (O'Neill 1998).

In the US, sexual harassment of women in the armed forces has been well documented and 'while it has always been a problem, sexual abuse, harassment and discrimination against women expanded enormously when the services decided to recruit large numbers of women and to integrate them with men' as the military became all-volunteer rather than draft-enlisted (O'Neill 1998: 61). Although the military became gender-integrated it remained male-dominated, and for some 'the fraternity of Naval and Marine airmen was being ruined', a 'fraternity' characterised by 'sexism, misogyny, sexual misconduct and discrimination' (ibid.: 64). A US Department of Defense survey identified 70 per cent of women and 30 per cent of men in active service had experienced sexual harassment in the prior 12 months (Antecol and Cobb-Clark 2001) and a Veterans Association survey estimated that half of female veterans experienced sexual harassment and a quarter experienced sexual assault during their military career (Skinner et al. 2000). A similar survey had earlier estimated that sexual assault while in the military was 20 times higher than in other government jobs (Murdoch and Nichol 1995). This is in sharp contrast to a highly proscriptive sexual conduct code, which forbids adultery, homosexuality and sexual relations between personnel, and which is sometimes implemented so vigorously that suspects are questioned about 'sexual performance, favourite positions and type of birth control ... to outsiders, the demands for intimate details sounded like sexual harassment' (O'Neill 1998: 67). Thus, strict regulation of sexual conduct from the centre of the institution is at odds with the lived experience of personnel in the field, in training centres and at the barracks; and policies from the top of the institutional hierarchy may be muted or transformed in their implementation by those at the top of their own local hierarchy. It is also suggestive that strict codes and potential for discipline after abuse has occurred need to be matched by prevention strategies in order to effectively change institutional behaviour norms, and promote safety.

IPV is also common for women in the US military, with around a quarter of serving women aged under 50 years experiencing IPV in the prior 12 months, of which half said that at least one incident has been life threatening (Murdoch and Nichol 1995). Violence in military families is gendered, with young boys at greater risk of physical abuse and young girls at greater risk of sexual abuse (Raiha and Soma 1997). Child mortality connected to military personnel is associated with prior physical abuse of the child and the perpetrator being his or her biological father (Lucas et al. 2002). These trends, women being abused by their partners, the over-representation of girls as victims of sexual abuse and the threat of early-life fatal abuse coming from within the family unit, mirror those in common society (Rentz et al. 2006); and are the reverse of the trends noted in the previous section on abuse by religious professionals.

In the UK in 1996, the Ministry of Defence responded to revelations of physically and sexually abusive initiations through changes to the Queen's Regulations for the Army, making unauthorised initiations illegal, and the report and investigation of which was placed under the auspice of the Royal Military Police (Wither 2004). A zero-tolerance policy has been introduced, supported by confidential telephone lines for advice and changes in reporting structures which have allowed complaints to be made outside of the chain of command. Physical abuse in the armed forces, through bullying and harassment, may be closer to inevitable as service personnel have to learn to adapt to high stress situations and training may be necessarily harsh. The overall rate of suicide in the armed forces is lower than in the general population, and lower in comparison to the suicide rates of the US military (Fear and Williamson 2003). However, the suicide rate of the youngest age group in the Army is higher than the other services and age groups, as well as higher than the equivalent general population group (ibid.), which may be indicative that vulnerable young adults, placed in stressful training situations may be traumatised and at additional risk of self-harm.

Peacekeeping forces have also been implicated in the abuse of displaced or war-stricken communities. Reports from the United Nations have identified that the presence of UN peacekeeping forces has been associated with the exchange of sex for money, food, jobs and an increase in child prostitution, both in refugee camps and in countries recovering from civil war, including Bosnia, Cambodia and Rwanda (UN 2005). This exploitation includes

> 'rape disguised as prostitution', in which [girls] were raped and given money or food afterwards to give the rape the appearance of a consensual transaction. Once young girls are in this situation, a situation of dependency is created which tends to result in a continued downward spiral of further prostitution, with its attendant violence, desperation, disease and further dependency.
>
> (UN 2005: 8)

The UN has further indentified a range of social–temporal–environmental factors that facilitate abuses, which include:

> the erosion of the social fabric because of the conflict, which results in a high number of children with little or no family support; a high level of extreme poverty; lack of income-generation possibilities; a high incidence of sexual violence against women and children during the civil conflict coupled with discrimination against women and girls, leading to a degree of local acceptance of violent and/or exploitative behaviour against them; and the lack of a well-functioning legal and judicial system, which creates an environment of de facto impunity.
>
> (United Nations 2005: 10)

In this way, a troubled community that most needs outside forces to be present is the least able to resist or respond defensively to misuses of the power that external agencies bring to it. Shortages of resources can contribute to a process whereby women and children become commodified and can be traded, and, in a traumatised and disrupted community, exploitation can be normalised and go unchallenged. Processes of depersonalisation and normalisation of abuse within militarised settings have also been suggested as explanations for the misconduct and abuses perpetrated on inmates at Abu Ghraib prison in Iraq (Department of Defense 2004; Titunik 2009). The next section considers abuses within prison settings further.

In this section it has been argued that abuse in the forms of sexual harassment and bullying is common in military life. Sexism and homophobia may be implicated in the underlying causes of some forms of harassment, as well as a need to 'toughen up' recruits as part of making troops ready for conflict. The authority and embodiment of (potential) aggression that characterises militaries and their personnel may be intrinsic qualities to their effectiveness that also act as abuse-promoting powers in unscrupulous and poorly controlled settings. Within conflict situations, women are particularly at risk of being victimised by the military, with rape being used as a strategy of war and as a strategy of exploitation in post-conflict areas. Inquiries have been called into the conduct of armed forces across all levels of activity, from training centres through to active service units, many of which have been perceived to lack transparency.

Prisons

This section will briefly consider abuse perpetrated in prison settings. As in the previous two sections, there is the possibility for '360 degree' harassment and assault: perpetrated by staff or inmates, against staff or inmates, vertically and horizontally within a hierarchy. As with military settings, a prison is supposed to be strictly administered with tough adherence to regulations and legitimate correctional punishments for those who offend. As with religious institutions, prisons are supposed to be safe places, with a high duty of care for the staff and inmates. However, arguably the power differentials between prison staff and prisoners are amplified, with the inmates intentionally and broadly disempowered through environmental confinement, revocation of fundamental societal privileges and institutionalised subordination to the penal system, with no immediate choice or power to withdraw or separate from the institutional setting. Perhaps unsurprisingly, there are high rates of abuse, exploitation and harassment within prisons, with routine or 'mundane' victimisation of assault, theft, intimidation and bullying (O'Donnell and Edgar 1998), as well as sexual violence and exploitation (Isaac et al. 2001).

Gender and ethnicity may be influential in patterns of abuse. Compared to male inmates who identified themselves as having been sexually abused in prison, female inmates are more likely to be abused by the staff (41 per cent compared to 8 per cent); however, more men than women reported being raped in prison (54 per cent compared to 28 per cent) (Struckman-Johnson and Struckman-Johnson 2006). Factors that influence victimisation of prisoners are related to individual and prison-level characteristics, so that ethnicity is important as the ethnicity of the victim but also as the proportion of ethnic minorities within the prison (Lahm 2009). The risk of being abused while in prison may be associated with the kind of person they are and the kind of offender they have been on the 'outside'; however, it is the prison staff and institution that retains the power to maintain conduct and safety within the prison setting. Prison staff have the dual responsibility for preventing abuse by guards as well as preventing and responding to abuses perpetrated by inmates, and as such, prison staff need to be specifically trained in non-abusive techniques of managing prisoners, as well as requiring training to identify and curb sexual assaults (Alarid 2000; Dumond 2000; Wolff et al. 2008). In addition to training, prison staff should be equipped to carry out high surveillance of inmates' interactions in order to implement zero-tolerance of abuse policies (Alarid 2000; Moster and Jeglic 2009). In line with the Delphi experts' conclusions discussed earlier, sexual and domestic violence offenders should have access to rehabilitation as part of their contact with the prison system, and should be assessed for aggravating issues, such as personality disorders or communication problems, as well as being assessed for their readiness and suitability for engaging in rehabilitative programmes to address their offending.

Healthcare and therapists

In the last of the four industries explored in this chapter, health and therapeutic professionals will be considered. Health and care professionals are widely accessed by the general population. For victims of sexual or domestic violence a healthcare provider can be a source of immediate medical help and also the first step to accessing services, advocacy, referrals for therapeutic treatment and support. Their role in identifying abuse and providing points of contact between victims and pathways to healing and intervention is essential. However, health and therapeutic industries are numerous, regulated to varying extents and often attract a high concentration of vulnerable people as clients. Accessible sympathy, attention and interaction may also be attractive to parts of the population seeking someone to harass, and health workers in acute settings often see the general population at their worst; stressed, uncertain, with high levels of intoxication, anxiety and distress, and easily provoked to angry outbursts. Security, administrative staff, nurses and doctors are all victims of violence in the workplace within healthcare settings (Yassi 1994), with physical, verbal and sexual abuse, threats, harassment and intimidation common throughout the NHS in spite of zero-tolerance policies (Gabe and Elston 2008).

Residents in medical training experience sexual harassment and a range of bigotry and abuse from superiors in the medical profession and from their patients. Female residents are more likely to experience sexual harassment than males (van Ineveld et al. 1996), findings that reflect patterns of harassment of female clergy members, discussed above. Also reflecting abuse within religious institutions, there is general public deference to the medical profession, with doctors exerting professional power over their patients. This makes mutual consent difficult to negotiate. If patients decide to report to authorities inappropriate sexual contact with their doctor, the power imbalance is sustained with medical professionals holding a better position within the complaints process, as well as having access to sensitive, and potentially discrediting, information about the victim (Rodgers 1995; Kendrick and Taylor 2000).

Outside of the main medical institutions, three factors contribute to sexual exploitation in health and care settings: insufficient regulation, inadequate training and definition of boundaries, and being a client of the mental health system. In the foreword to the Protection of Vulnerable Adults guidelines, it is asserted that harm caused to adults in health and social care settings is usually not due to 'malice' but to insufficient professional capabilities (DH 2004a: 4). Screening out of workers with a history of neglectful, harmful or abusive practices, increased training and better knowledge of boundaries within health and care settings are advocated. Across the health industry 'there are a substantial number of people providing health and social care whose behaviour is unregulated, and where there are no mechanisms for bringing a complaint against them unless their behaviour could be defined as criminal' (Williams and Nash 2001: 367). Harm to clients can occur both intentionally, through physical and sexual abuse, and unintentionally through mismanagement of professional boundaries. For many organisations within the health field, the lack of documented ethical codes of conduct, robust complaints procedures and institutional accountability are abuse-promoting factors (POPAN 2004). Where clients seek to make a complaint about abuse or misconduct, they frequently experience that the 'process of formally complaining is more legalistic, very demanding, and often damaging, with outcomes that are rarely satisfying' (Williams and Nash 2001: 363). Across the health industries, there are abuse-prevention needs of providing better training and clearer boundaries for staff, as well as better information to be made available to clients about professional boundaries and grievance procedures to make patients less vulnerable in one-to-one interactions with health and care staff. Alongside this, instances of abuse need to be better managed, with an independent complaints body that can withdraw practitioners from the field when complaints of sexual exploitation or abuse are upheld: ethical codes should be enforced and enforceable and made clear to practitioners and clients (POPAN 2004; Williams and Nash 2001).

Patients/clients in the mental health field may be at greater risk of exploitation, especially when staying on psychiatric inpatient wards (Cole et al.

2003). One in five psychiatric inpatient wards have in their records confirmed sexual interactions between staff and patients in the prior two years, which represents both a failure to prevent exploitation as well as instances of sexual assault (Kumar 2000). Psychiatrists under-report abuses when they are disclosed; for example, in a survey 65 per cent reported treating patients who disclosed having previous sexual contact with a therapist, but only 8 per cent of those cases were reported (ibid.). In the primary health sector, patients with complex mental-health needs are generally underserved, with the primary care system failing to compensate for communication and/or cognitive impairments when present. Patients/clients with mental health needs may be less able to assert their rights, and when going through a complaints process they may be less credible (for example if they have been previously diagnosed with delusions) or less sympathetic (for example if they have a history of violence) (ibid.).

There have been many similarities between this section and the previous three: the need for improvements in training, regulation and accountability, and the power imbalance between staff and clients, brought about in part by social deference to the profession and in part by the dependency of the clients on the professional for help. Advocates in the field have outlined clear directions for improvements in practice that would support abuse-prevention and redress strategies. In the final piece of research literature presented here, a comparison was sought between survivors of medical, mental health or clergy professional exploitation and abuse (Disch and Avery 2001).

Comparing adult respondents who had been abused by a medical, mental health or religious professional during their lifetime, survivors were found to have similar high rates of previous physical and/or childhood sexual abuse. Differences between the sectors emerged in offending patterns. There was an increasing median age at first instance of abuse across professions, with abuse by a medical professional generally initiated earlier than abuse by clergy, which in turn was generally earlier than abuse by a mental health professional. This seems consistent with a typical life trajectory and exposure to or contact with the different services. There were also differences in the length of abuse, increasing from medical, to clergy, to mental health-based abuses, so that overall medical and clergy abuses tended to occur at a younger age, and mental health sector abuse tended to last longer. When respondents reported the consequences and effects of their abuse experiences, medical abuse survivors were more likely to be unable to think about parts of the abuse or have panic attacks, and scored highest on 10 out of 15 subscales of distress. This is indicative that abuse by medical practitioners needs to be taken as seriously as other sectors, and that age at initiation and length of abuse are not necessarily good predictors of long-term sequelae of abuse for all sectors. The potential for differences between sectors, both in terms of the structure and emergence of abuse, as well as the experience and effects of abuse, is important to consider in the following conclusions, where points of general principle are identified.

Conclusions

Abuse by professionals is pervasive across the sectors considered in this chapter, with abuse being multi-directional, mostly directed towards subordinates or clients, but also between peers. Across the sectors there emerges a common trope comparing abuse by professionals to hunting in commentaries about power inequalities between the general population and the profession. Kelly refers to an 'open season' on women during wartime (2000: 60); Kluft refers to incest survivors seeking psychotherapy as 'sitting ducks' (1990: 90); Disch and Avery refer to 'hunters' and 'prey' in their examination of survivors from the fields of health and religious institutions (2001: 216).

The societal and contextual setting of professions and sectors is important and the chapter concludes with a five-factor model of the underlying determinants of professions which facilitate abuse and generate the power that facilitates abuses at the levels of both the individual and profession.

1 Superiority from the population masses

First, the profession is seen as somehow set apart from the rest of the population. For the clergy this was most clearly articulated by the notion of clericalism, but there are similar principles in the social deference to doctors and in the training of military recruits into the elite armed forces. For prison staff, their superiority over the imprisoned population is part of their job role.

2 Hierarchical

Secondly, the profession has an internal hierarchy, which privileges particular views and behaviours and passes over others, encouraging compliance with the professional identity. The hierarchy also allows for professional norms to be set, regulated and reproduced at intermediate levels, offering social control within the institution and allowing power to accumulate at interim points, progressing towards the top. The notion of 'our own' or 'us' is reinforced. This is observed in career paths and increasing rank conferred to more established members of the profession.

3 Identity conferred by the institution and carried outside of the institutional setting

Thirdly, there is a giving up of part of one's individual identity to the profession, which is returned by the conferring of professional identity that lasts outside of the professional setting, for example in the titles of Father, Sister, Doctor, Colonel, etc.

4 Exceptionalism

Fourthly, the professional role grants the individual some exception from the regulations and restrictions placed on the rest of the population. Priests can withhold information if it was shared under the secrecy of confession without it being labelled contempt of court; surgeons can cut sedated patients open without it being labelled a grievous bodily assault; soldiers can shoot their opponents without it being labelled murder; prison staff can lock up the prison without it being labelled kidnapping.

5 Responsibility for fixing problems

Fifthly, the professional is asked to fix problems on behalf of the rest of the population, which creates some dependency on that profession, for example doctors are conduits to healthcare and prescriptions, priests are conduits to absolution and god's teachings, the army is asked to defend the country, prison officers are asked to keep prisons peaceful and secure.

In this model, prison staff fit the least well, as their authority and hierarchy are localised to their work environment, whereas clergy and the military fit most closely, with the health field decreasingly fitting less well as distance increases away from traditional medical services. The military and the clergy share additional similarities, including enforced sexuality as enforced heterosexuality for the military and celibacy for the clergy (though not outside of the Catholic clergy). For the military and non-Catholic clergy, the profession is male-dominated, with the recent introduction of women to the institution or to its higher ranks. Perhaps the most important similarities between the sectors are the corroborated accusations of a cover-up of abuses; for example, the Commission to Inquire into Child Abuse (2009) and Taguba report (US Department of Defense 2004), as well as findings from research papers that around one in three people who report their abuse to authorities are discredited or harassed (Disch and Avery 2001); and the need at any point in the last 20 years to launch a 'zero-tolerance' policy in response to emerging scandals. The failure of informal or discretionary policies and subsequent introduction of a zero-tolerance approach is a likely indicator that underlying abuse-promoting power or practices exist within an institution.

Implications for practice are therefore: recognise the potential power that is held within your profession and how that can facilitate abuse; ensure that staff are trained to fulfil their own responsibility for offering safe, well-boundaried practice and also trained to identify and respond appropriately to incidents of misconduct and abuse; manage social deference responsibly and balance it with a strong commitment to the equitable treatment of disadvantaged and vulnerable clients or co-workers; provide and adhere to clear, easy to understand and easily available codes of conduct; work to uphold an ethical code and remove workers who demonstrate misconduct; endorse institutional practices that seek historical victims of abuse and work towards redress, and develop good practice that respects existing victims.

Part IV

Tackling sexual and domestic violence and abuse

Moving towards improved prevention and early intervention

The final part of this book turns to consider what more needs to be done to tackle domestic and sexual violence and abuse, and to achieve greater success in preventing violence and abuse and in responding through earlier intervention to ensure consequences are minimised. The single chapter in this part summarises the major messages from the earlier parts of the book. From these conclusions it is possible to draw out the implications for improving outcomes for individuals through: policy development; service and practice improvement; and lastly the needs for further research. The chapter highlights a number of important overarching and underlying principles: the importance of hope and recovery in the treatment of victims and abusers; the need to understand and address the gendered nature of domestic and sexual violence and abuse; domestic and sexual violence and abuse as everyone's responsibility – the core business of all health, mental health and other relevant services across sectors; and finally, the importance of addressing health inequalities and social exclusion.

10 Conclusions and implications for research, policy and practice

Within the Press release that launched the VVAPP programme in November 2006, Professor Louis Appleby, National Director for Mental Health said:

> Childhood physical, emotional and sexual abuse and neglect, and domestic violence can have long-lasting, devastating effects on the mental health and well-being of those who are victimised. Developing effective preventative and therapeutic interventions is an important part of the mental health modernisation programme.

While Professor David Colin-Thome, National Director of Primary Care acknowledged:

> I know that we GPs are not always fully equipped and supported to identify and respond to the needs of domestic abuse, or rape or childhood sexual abuse. This work should help to increase awareness and understanding and improve the care provided.

This book summarises the steps that need to be taken to respond to the analysis encapsulated in these two quotes. It has covered an enormous breadth of material. Taking a life-course approach, it has situated the findings from a major study of the views of experts by profession and experts by experiences, and other studies of the pathways that individual victims/survivors have traced through services in their journeys towards healing, within the research evidence accumulated from decades of studies into the epidemiology of violence and abuse, and primary, secondary and tertiary interventions in this field. The book has focused on sexual and domestic violence and abuse; however, it has emphasised the need to see these as inherently situated within social structures nested from the local up to the global level – a socio-ecological framework was introduced in Chapter 2 and used throughout. These social structures interact differently to influence individuals' experiences according to characteristics such as age, gender, sexuality, ethnicity and (dis)ability.

Chapter 2 emphasised the value base that the Delphi experts considered important for practice, with a human rights/equalities framework regarded as an essential basis for policy and practice, this was re-emphasised through-out the contributions in Part III of the book on addressing inequalities. Chapter 2 also emphasised the importance of practice guidelines and codes of professional conduct. While there was no consensus about whether these needed to be distinct sets for different areas of practice/professions or not, there was a clear need for survivors to be made aware of the existence of these, and how to raise any concerns they might have. The need for regular updating of all sets of guidelines and for systems for assuring adherence were also strongly emphasised.

Although, as chapters throughout the book have emphasised, knowledge is not complete, enough is known to clearly set out what needs to be done and how to achieve it. This is not to say, however, that making the required changes will be easy. A number of major challenges remain. First and fore-most is achieving the necessary political will to support, and resource, the relevant services and initiatives.

As the next section explores, changes are necessary throughout all sectors of society in order to achieve the necessary whole of system/society implemen-tation to address violence and abuse adequately. Political will is necessary, not just in the short term, but into the medium and long term, as the necessary changes and implementation of a public health prevention framework cannot be achieved in the short lifetimes of single governments. A major component in what is necessary is effective interagency collaboration, based on clear understanding of the complementary roles that different agencies have to play within an overall public health framework, and clear protocols to permit information and resource sharing. The case studies presented throughout the book and the analysis presented in Chapter 7 demonstrated very clearly the importance of such collaboration.

Success will not be complete, however, without breaking through the silence and shame that still cloaks much violence and abuse; silence and shame on the behalf of the victims or survivors who fear condemnation and blame from those individuals and agencies who should provide support and services, and silence and shame on the behalf of perpetrators who wish to hide their responsibility for their acts and actions and refuse the possibility of change. This requires a major change in attitudes in society, from a view that sees violence and abuse as perpetrated by the evil stranger to views that see vio-lence and abuse as things that need to be tackled throughout the fabric of society, in private as well as public spheres, as something that individuals need to address within themselves. As the foundation for this change, recognition of the centrality of human rights, and respect for diversity and difference, are essential to addressing the needs of both victims/survivors and perpetrators.

The remainder of this chapter is presented in three sections, the first of these summarises the public health prevention framework that represents the summation of what has been discussed in Chapters 2 to 9. A second section then examines the key conclusions in terms of improving outcomes for individuals, focusing in turn on policy development, service and practice improvement and finally on further research needs. The chapter finishes by discussing important principles underpinning this work.

A public health prevention framework

The book has emphasised that a public health approach is required to respond to this major public health problem. Figure 10.1 summarises the public health prevention framework that represents the summation of Chapters 2 to 9. The Delphi experts overwhelmingly emphasised the importance of a public health approach to prevention, first and foremost aimed at changing societal attitudes to violence and abuse. The later chapters of the book presented the research evidence that underpins this approach and identified some key components.

Greater awareness among the general public about sexual and domestic violence and abuse is important. Public awareness campaigns need to stress

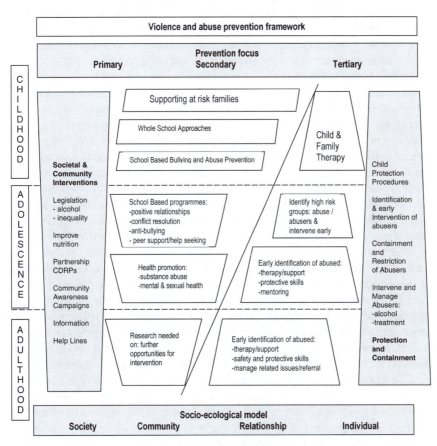

Figure 10.1 A framework for responding to violence and abuse.

Source: Adapted and updated from Nurse (2006), used with permission.

personal responsibilities and rights, and there needs to be careful work with the media to try and ensure that sensational coverage (which attracts good audiences) does not overshadow the informational and educational content that those who are quietly or secretly living with memories prior to disclosure need. Other important interventions at societal or community level include legislation and the provision of helplines. Within the UK, Crime and Disorder Reduction Partnerships (CDRPs) potentially have a key role in leading the partnership effort that is necessary, but issues around confidentiality and information sharing will need to be resolved for their full potential to be realised.

Awareness and information sessions need to be provided in schools as part of the Personal, Social and Health Education curriculum. Sexual and domestic violence and abuse need to be made priority issues for education services, with additional support for teachers who are supporting pupils who disclose.

The need for application of a basic public health model (of identifying risk factors and strengthening protective factors in the individual, the family, the community and society within various age bands) has been emphasised. Prevention needs to be approached as any other major public health campaign, with appropriate components for primary, secondary and tertiary prevention; these components are summarised in Figure 10.1.

Children and young people are most likely to be safe and keep safe if they: understand their right to be safe, have been helped to develop the confidence to speak out if they feel danger, or don't like what is happening; have a secure base within a family or substitute family; there is at least one adult they can talk to. Therefore building children's self-esteem and self-worth and listening to and taking them seriously should be at the core of all universal services and should be part of a strategy in, say, PHSE for equipping children to grow safely and healthily, with an understanding of healthy relationships and consent. This needs to be developed through adolescence into knowledge and understanding about safe dating. Education of learning-disabled people about sexual activity and relationships is also required.

The issues of lack of funding, lack of political will, lack of priority and lack of public visibility and the need for societal-wide action come through in every single programme area – along with support for a broad public health approach and the need for an integrated high-profile national strategy (with some differences about the extent to which integration is possible/ desirable). Policy-makers need to resist the temptation to impose unitary solutions to the huge diversity of different situations and recognise that the keys to successful policies are likely to be sensitivity and flexibility.

The current lack of joined-up approach at national level needs to be addressed through a comprehensive national strategy that recognises the need for action in all sectors of society. Three particular components are particularly important. The need for widespread change in public attitudes and knowledge about the extent and nature of abuse had already been mentioned, but here it is important to keep an appropriate balance between the coverage of 'stranger danger' and abuse by known and trusted adults, with recognition that men are also victims/survivors of sexual violence and abuse. There is a need for government departments to work with the media to give clear messages that people can recognise and take appropriate action about abusive behaviours. Second is the need to challenge the silence about abuse and sexual abuse.

There is also a need to challenge the problem of abuse not being seen as relevant in NHS settings, e.g. not a 'mental health' issue. This relates to services still being organised around diagnostic categories and medical models of care where links are not made between experience of abuse and presenting distress or 'symptoms'. Once a person has a diagnostic label (e.g. ADHD, Personality Disorder', OCD, etc.) all too often it is assumed that there is no need to ask any more questions; this inhibits disclosure and addressing the underlying needs in favour of mere symptom management.

In terms of funding, the need for long-term funding for all different sectors is vital. Funding for the NGO sector on a long-term rather than short-term basis, thereby retaining NGO expertise, is particularly important since not all victims/survivors feel safe to access statutory sector services (assuming that such services exist).

Throughout all sectors of society, organisations need to proactively 'model' non-abusive and empowering behaviours, and workplace bullying and harassment policies have an important role to play here.

A less punitive and more therapeutic approach is required towards the perpetrators, who must be treated firmly and appropriately and not let off or cautioned. Adequate resources to be able to offer and strongly encourage the uptake of treatment must be available. There must be zero-tolerance of violent and abusive behaviour. Other important components of service provision include an increase in the availability of advice to those who know they have a sexual interest in children, such as confidential free phone numbers and a need to have facilities available for those who have no criminal record but who are concerned about their behaviour/desires. Also relevant here are restrictions in availability of pornographic material, given the role of such material in increased risk of developing pro-rape attitudes, beliefs and behaviours, and committing sexual offences (Itzin et al. 2007).

Improving outcomes for individuals

Therapy has three stages – building trust, working through and letting go. Trust takes time to establish. The therapist needs to be consistent in approach and clear about boundaries. Timing is important, sessions must begin and end on time. The demeanour of the therapist must be consistent. Low self-esteem means that every step is a hurdle to be overcome – we simply do not believe that we are worth people's attention. Therefore the therapist needs to be prepared to be tested by the survivors who will expect to be rejected and will try to ensure that rejection occurs. In my own case this initial stage took many sessions as I worked through my suspicions of my therapist's intentions, motivation and tried to break down the boundaries. He remained empathetic but firm. During the working through stage the survivor will have leant that the therapist is trustworthy (although this does not mean that the strategies described above will not re-occur during difficult sessions). Low self-esteem continues to be problematic and with many survivors, such as myself, it is never solved entirely. We reach a position where we know we are not 'bad' but can feel 'bad' at times. This difference between cognitive and affective is important when working with survivors. Cognition is paramount. Therapists need to ensure that the survivor understands the process of therapy and be given time to reflect on the work being done. This emphasis on the survivor knowing why the work is being done as it is and what is happening, reduces the risk of a power imbalance in the therapy room. In my own case this took several years while I talked about my abuse for the first time. These sessions were often fraught with difficulties and my therapist was sensitive to the fact that I had to drive home, stopping the session early so I could 'return to my adult self' for a few minutes before leaving. He worked in such a way that I understood what was happening and taught me how to apply this knowledge away from therapy sessions so I could cope with the frightening situation I found myself in. He also insisted that I could manage, something that I did not believe initially but learnt that I was more capable of looking after myself than I thought. This insistence that I could succeed if I struggled with the work of therapy was an important factor in my healing.

(Delphi expert, talking about healing from childhood sexual abuse)

Policy development and service and practice improvement

Diversity, inclusion, equal treatment and basic human rights principles were strongly suggested as fundamentally important, suggesting that a human rights/equalities framework was a required basis for policy and practice, with explicit attention to gender, sexuality, ethnicity, and disability within this. A second overarching theme was the notion of the importance of a victim/survivor-centred approach (associated with characteristics such as empowerment, giving control and choice to victims/survivors); this was suggested, by some, to include choice for victims/survivors in terms of the gender, sexuality and age of the person they work with.

As the quote that opened this section emphasised, belief in possibility of healing is vital for those who would work as healers, coupled with an appropriate humility that their role is as a facilitator. The counterpart of this for those who work with perpetrators is the belief that their change is possible and lies within their control.

A lack of availability of resources is the key obstacle to realising the potential for making a significant difference to the lives of those who have experienced violence and abuse. All too often, individuals suffer in a form of postcode lottery as to whether access to therapeutic services is achieved in a timely fashion.

Further research

As has been emphasised above, research has given us insight into a variety of different approaches that work in terms of providing for positive outcomes. The amount of evidence from well-designed, well-executed studies is still low in some cases (below what some sets of criteria regard as sufficient). To a great extent this reflects the limitations on available research funding – particularly for studies with the long follow-up periods necessary to allow for healing of complex, long-lasting and multi-faceted abuse. As has been emphasised earlier in this book, an absence of evidence is not the same as evidence of absence. Further research is necessary to increase the amount and quality of evidence available, and to enable us to better understand how to tailor a package of services and responses to the needs of particular individuals.

Earlier chapters in the book have identified issues where no clear research evidence exists and where Delphi experts hold diverging views. These indicate areas that would benefit from future research attention to understand better the task of tailoring appropriate therapeutic interventions to the specifics of each individual's history and experience.

Another need is better understanding of what promotes and facilitates resilience in individuals, families and communities. Research that investigates this is still all too rare, although there are some signs that this is beginning to change. For example, Thomas and Hall (2008) describe a narrative study of thriving adult female survivors of child abuse, which identifies a wide range of different turning points and their role in women's life trajectories.

Overarching principles

Hope and recovery

The importance of hope and recovery in the treatment of both victims/survivors and abusers cannot be overestimated. Here, the clear view of the therapist that healing and change are possible has an important part to play. Just as educational research has taught us that the expectations of teachers about individual pupils' chances of success or failure influences those pupils' educational outcomes, so expectations of therapists can influence outcomes for clients.

Addressing the gendered nature of domestic and sexual violence and abuse

Chapter 6 above examined the gendering of interpersonal violence and abuse; and the implications of sexuality for the experience of interpersonal violence and abuse by heterosexual, lesbian and gay individuals. While the literature on violence and abuse often considers gender and sexuality as separate issues and phenomena, processes of gendering and issues related to sexuality are by no means discrete, and Chapter 6 explored some of the overlaps, links and implications of difference. Gender is of crucial importance to understanding the impact of interpersonal violence and abuse on individuals, and understanding what may work in overcoming victimisation (Itzin 2000a). At the same time, sexuality creates different experiences and outcomes. The social construction of masculinity, as embodied in heterosexual men, helps to explain, for instance, domestic violence as the exertion of power and control by men over women in intimate relationships within contexts of gender inequality (Hester 2004). In same-sex relationships gender is not as prominent in positioning individuals within relationships and in interactions and constructions of power and violence. There is, however, still evidence of gendered norms impacting on experiences and outcomes of violence and abuse for lesbians and gay men (Hester and Donovan 2009).

The contentious issue of men as victims of domestic violence and abuse and women as perpetrators has dominated the past decade, and in particular the use of the CTS (Conflict Tactics Scale) in producing findings of 'symmetry' between women and men as perpetrators and men more than women as victims (Archer 2000). However, the use of CTSs to measure IPV is problematic, as a result of methodological flaws in the instrument. The nature of the problem with CTSs requires explanation because of the perverse effects their use has had on public policy in the US, in particular, but increasingly in the UK and Europe.

The problem lies in the CTS's use of act-based measures without examination of context in terms of physical or social power differentials. This has led Archer (2000) to conclude that measured by the CTS, men's and women's use of acts is symmetrical, but the consequences are not symmetric. Dobash and Dobash (2004) have offered a more sophisticated critique. The first issue is the use of ambiguous items, for example, in one version of the CTS, men and women were asked if they had ever 'thrown an object at your partner', when it is clear that throwing a lamp at a partner is very different from throwing a pillow. A second issue is that of multiple or compound items, for example: 'hit or tried to hit your partner with something', when actually hitting a partner is very different from trying to hit a partner. This type of act-based approach makes no distinction between the physical impact/consequences of a slap delivered by a slight, small woman with a blow delivered by a heavier, stronger, taller man.

In their paper, Dobash and Dobash identify an additional problem with act-based measures: that the usual scoring methods are such that it is only necessary for a man or a woman to indicate that they have committed one single act on the list in order to be defined as violent. This means that those who have perpetrated several violent acts (no matter how serious) and those who have reported committing only one act (no matter how trivial) are both defined as violent. Thus the woman who admits that she tried to hit her partner is equated with the man who reports beating his partner up: both are deemed to be violent and it is concluded that there is symmetry in their use of violence. They identify another problem as 'the conflation of violence (physical and sexual acts) with other non-violent acts of abuse (shouting, name-calling etc.)' (p. 331). The danger is that researchers may conclude that women are just as violent as men when what may, in fact, be under discussion is men's acts of physical and sexual violence and women's acts of arguing or shouting. From their own research with men convicted of violence and their partners, using a context-specific method, Dobash and Dobash found that serious intimate partner violence is asymmetrical, with men usually violent to women. Johnson's (2008) analysis is pertinent here; he criticises CTSs for failing to distinguish between the different types of domestic violence – that which involves coercive control (IPA in the terms defined in Chapter 1 and 'intimate terrorism' in Johnson's terms) and that which does not – situational couple violence in Johnson's terms.

In later chapters in Part 3, the importance of gender was also illustrated. Chapter 7 showed how the intersection of gender, race and culture produce specific risks of violence and abuse for different black and minority ethnic populations. As Chapter 8 showed, the experiences of disabled people are also shaped by gender as well as ethnicity, as the different case studies described amply illustrate. Finally, in Chapter 9, intersections of gender and profession again produce particular patterns of risk and experience.

Sexual and domestic violence and abuse as everyone's responsibility

One of the major challenges to achieving appropriate responses to sexual and domestic violence and abuse within the health sector has been the mistaken perception that these are not health issues, that they are social problems. The enormous wealth of evidence about the serious short-, medium- and long-term health effects for violence and abuse that Chapters 2 to 6 in this book have summarised demonstrate that this mistaken belief must be firmly countered by ensuring that all health professionals, as a part of their basic, pre-registration training, are introduced to the basic epidemiology of violence and abuse and its health consequences. Asking about experience of violence and abuse needs to become an integral part of the basic history-taking that is expected wherever any of the sign/symptoms that are associated with violence and abuse occur. Without this, important opportunities for prevention and early intervention will be lost.

But tackling violence and abuse is the business of not only the health sector – it needs to be part of the core business of all health, mental health and other relevant services across all sectors. As this book has illustrated throughout, especially in the various case studies presented and in particular the section by Hanmer in Chapter 7.2, multi-agency approaches are necessary for responding to and providing interventions for domestic and sexual violence. Sharing information between agencies is important for multi-agency work, but issues of confidentiality and data protection define and limit the sorts of information that may be shared and with whom, and providing appropriate protocols in this area remains a challenge for the future. Appropriate primary prevention work aimed at changing attitudes to violence and abuse needs to take place across all sectors in a coordinated fashion for maximum effect. In terms of funding, the need for long-term funding for all different sectors and in particular retaining NGO expertise was emphasised, since all not all victims/survivors feel safe to access statutory sector services (assuming that such services exist).

Addressing health inequalities and social exclusion

As various parts of the book have emphasised, the health consequences of violence and abuse are enormous; this is one of the reasons that the issue is such a public health priority. The implementation of an appropriate framework to tackle violence and abuse will make a vitally important contribution to the reduction of health inequalities.

The book has also discussed the stigma and shame that attends the experience of domestic and sexual violence and abuse, and how this reinforces the negative effects of violence and abuse, interferes with the processes of seeking appropriate help and support, and can maintain those who have experienced violence and abuse in states of social isolation and social exclusion (see also Taket et al. 2009 for an amplification of these arguments).

In order to fully address the challenge of the social exclusion of those who have experienced domestic and sexual violence and abuse, widespread societal change in terms of attitudes to violence and abuse is necessary, overturning the different stereotypes that place the blame and shame on the victims, and recognising the operation of coercive control for what it is, an abuse of an individual's basic human rights.

Human rights and social justice in domestic and sexual violence and abuse

Domestic and sexual violence and abuse represent a violation of the basic human rights of victims/survivors. Through the exercise of coercive control on the part of the abuser, the rights of victims/survivors to live in freedom and safety, to autonomy and self-determination are compromised, often severely, and with short-, medium- and long-term consequences to health and well-being. This provides a strong mandate for supporting the implementation of policies and practice to respond to domestic and sexual violence and abuse through early intervention and prevention. Throughout this book, it has been emphasised that a human rights framework that seeks to address rights violations and promote social justice offers a strong foundation for progress in the future.

Looking forward to looking back

> All abuse occurs from an absence of love for self and others. The essence of our humanity is love, which is an unlimited and free resource that resides within us all. It is time that we, as individuals and as a society found the courage and commitment to reawaken to and manifest that love. For love does not hurt, love does not judge. Re-connect with the love within, then abuse will not occur. Love empowers. Fear does not exist where there is love. … Professionals cannot share what they deny/repress within themselves. A complete change of attitude and approach from one of judgement, fear and indifference to one of professional objectivity combined with love and detached compassion. We live in a society in which individuals have judged themselves not worthy of their own love and therefore do not value themselves. If we do not love and value ourselves then we cannot love and value others nor respond effectively to their needs. When children are judged unworthy of love/live with criticism, abuse, etc., then they internalise those judgements and accept them as their own, this causes deep emotional pain which can be anaesthetised through drugs, drink etc. and/or manifests as depressions/rage. This is the source of abuse, mental illness etc. We need to address the fundamental cause of the mental illness within society, the absence of love through judgement and not continue to react to the symptoms.
>
> (Delphi expert)

To finish, it is useful to consider the question of what might be found in a future where the public health issue represented by sexual and domestic violence and abuse had been successfully tackled. This would be a future where every child and young person, regardless of gender, ethnicity, religion, class, sexuality or ability, believed in their right to nurturing and loving care, and understood their right to make their wishes clear, and could count on those wishes being heard, understood and supported by their family, community and the wider society. All individuals would be equipped with skills and understanding about their own worth as individuals and about the creation and maintenance of healthy relationships, both intimate and friendship. Service agencies would work to support the creation of healthy relationships and the healing of those where something had gone wrong, but, owing to the growth in skills and understanding throughout society, residual demand for services would be small. Research would have filled in some of the gaps outlined above, so that it is better understood how to support and facilitate resilience in individuals, families and communities, and to tailor interventions and services to the particular needs of individuals.

Appendix 1
UK Government policy initiatives in relation to violence and abuse

This list covers Department of Health policy documents which include domestic and sexual violence and abuse, and cross-government policy documents which include the role of the Department of Health in addressing these issues.

Mental health

- *Mental Health National Service Framework (DH 1999)* – highlights the 'association between child sexual and other abuse and domestic violence with mental illness and personality disorder'.
- *National Suicide Prevention Strategy (DH 2002a)* – includes 'promoting the mental health of victims and survivors of abuse, including child sexual abuse' with a focus on self-harm.
- *Women's Mental Health Strategy – Into the Mainstream (DH 2002b)* and *Implementation Guide – Mainstreaming Gender and Women's Mental Health (DH 2003)* – has a strong focus on child sexual abuse, rape and sexual assault and domestic violence as causal factors in mental illness for women and propose these become core issues in mental health services.
- *Mental Health Trusts Collaboration Project (MHTCP) routine enquiry pilots (2006–2008)* – evaluation report (McNeish and Scott 2008) providing guidance to mental health services based on national pilots introducing routine questions about child sexual abuse in assessments and treatment incorporated into care planning under the Care Programme Approach.
- *Delivering Race Equality in Mental Health Care (DH 2005a)* – includes the effects of domestic violence and child sexual abuse on mental health.

Children

- *National Service Framework for Children Young People and Maternity (DH and DES 2004)* – states that 'the abuse of a child – physically, emotionally or sexually – or neglect and domestic violence can have a serious impact on all aspects of the child's health, development and well-being which can last throughout adulthood, with immediate and longer term impact ... including anxiety, depression, substance misuse, eating disorders and self-destructive behaviours.'

- *Working Together to Safeguard Children: A Guide to Inter-Agency Working to Safeguard and Promote the Welfare of Children (HM Government 2006)* – includes a chapter on the role of health services in identifying and responding to the needs of abused children.

- *Chapter 6.7 of Working Together to Safeguard Children: A guide to interagency working to safeguard and promote the welfare of children (HM Government 2006)* – sets out clear policy which covers paedophile abuse, organised abuse involving families and communities, organised abuse involving rituals, and organisational abuse (using an institutional framework or position of authority).

- *Staying Safe (DCSF 2008b)* – sets out a detailed action plan for 2008–2011. It includes children who experience child sexual and other abuse as well as sexual exploitation and highlights the role of therapeutic and preventive interventions in responding to abuse.

- *Framework for the Assessment of Children in Need and their Families (Appendix 2 in HM Government 2006)* – provides the teams to identify children and families in need of early therapeutic, preventive and supportive interventions.

Public health

- *Public Health White Paper Choosing Health (DH 2004b)* – identifies child physical, emotional and sexual abuse and neglect and domestic violence as public health issues to be addressed through a cross-government strategy for tackling the health and mental health effects associated with this.

- *Public Health White Paper Delivery Plan (DH 2005c)* – includes 'the joint DH and HO initiatives to develop SARCs nationally, including services for children and adolescents, and improving the quality of patient experience for victims of domestic violence through the joint DH, HO and NIMHE violence and abuse programme'.

Social exclusion

- *Child Poverty Review (HM Treasury 2004)* – identifies 'the effects of child sexual abuse and domestic violence on children' as being 'associated with an increased lifetime prevalence of mental illness' and with 'mental health problems in childhood'.

- *Social Exclusion Unit Report on 'Mental Health and Social Exclusion' (2004)* – identifies 'victims of abuse – specifically those who have been sexually abused in childhood and adult victims of domestic violence as amongst those who often experience mental health problems'.

Domestic violence and abuse

- *Responding to Domestic Abuse: A Handbook for Health Professionals (DH 2005b)* – advises services and professionals on how to identify and respond to the needs of those experiencing domestic violence and the introduction of routine enquiry in ante-natal and other health services.
- *Responding to Domestic Abuse: Training Manual (DH and HO 2006)* – commissioned by the VVAPP and developed with the National Domestic Violence Practitioners Reference Group.
- *National Domestic Violence Delivery Plan (HO 2009a)* – produced annually since 2005 setting objectives for implementation of government legislation and policy on domestic violence and abuse.
- *Violence Against Women and Girls (HO 2009b)* – draws together the evidence of harm to women and girls to include domestic violence and abuse, childhood sexual abuse, adult rape and sexual assault, pornography, prostitution and trafficking.

Adult rape and child sexual abuse

- *Cross-Government Sexual Violence and Abuse Action Plan (HM Government 2007)* – contains a section on 'Support and Health Services' for children, adolescents and adults with the objective of increasing access to support and health services for victims of sexual violence and childhood sexual abuse through a combination of NHS services, voluntary sector services and Sexual Assault Referral Centres (SARCs). The section on 'Prevention' includes young people who sexually abuse and adult sex offenders.
- *A Resource for Developing Sexual Assault Referral Centres (SARCs) (DH et al. 2009)* – superseding previous guidance, this deals with the development of joint police, health and voluntary sector-run centres to provide support and counselling and forensic medical services for victims of rape and sexual assault. It sets out the key elements of a service for child victims of rape or sexual assault presenting to SARCs, as well as for adult victims/survivors.

Prostitution, pornography and trafficking

- *Consultation on the Possession of Extreme Pornographic Material (HO 2005b)* – proposed creating a new offence of simple possession of extreme pornographic material available on the internet and otherwise uncontrollable by existing legislation.
- *A Coordinated Prostitution Strategy and a Summary of Responses to Paying the Price (HO 2006)* – includes the role of health services providing outreach, sexual health services and drugs and alcohol interventions in supporting women to exit prostitution.

- *UK Action Plan on Human Trafficking (HO 2007b)* – covers children, adolescents and adults, the role of the DH safeguarding children, Child and Adolescent Mental Health Services (CAMHS) and VVAPP programmes in identifying and responding to their needs.
- *Safeguarding Children from Sexual Exploitation (DCSF 2007a)* – includes the health service role in identifying and responding to the needs of children sexually exploited through prostitution, pornography and trafficking.
- *Safeguarding Children Who May Have Been Trafficked (DCSF 2007b)* – includes guidance for 'practitioners on identifying signs of abuse and trafficking' in A&E, walk-in centres, minor injury units, GUM clinics, sexual health services, community contraceptive services, GPs, primary care trusts and school nurses'.

Sex offenders

- *Whittle et al (2006) The needs and effective treatment of young people who sexually abuse* – published as best practice guidance by Department of Health and Home Office.
- *Review of the Protection of Children from Sex Offenders (HO 2007a)* – supports the provision of community interventions with those at risk of new or continued offending creating the opportunity to provide community preventive interventions with familial sexual abusers in addition to the Sex Offender Treatment Programmes (SOTP) provided by the Prison Service.

Learning disabilities

- *Valuing People with Learning Disabilities: a new strategy for learning disabilities for the 21st century (DH 2001)* – emphasises that 'people with learning disabilities are entitled to at least the same level of support and protection from abuse and harm as other citizens'.
- *No Secrets – Guidance on Services for Vulnerable Adults (DH and HO 2000)* – guidance on implementing multi-agency policies and procedures with physical and learning disabled and older people who 'may be unable to protect [themselves] from significant harm or exploitation including physical abuse including physical abuse (hitting, slapping, pushing, kicking, misuse of medication) and sexual abuse (rape and sexual assault or sexual acts) to which the vulnerable adult has not consented, or could not consent or was pressured into consenting'.
- *Valuing People Now: a new three-year strategy for people with learning disabilities – making it happen for everyone (HM Government 2009)* – updates 2001 guidance with a section on 'Being Safe in the Community and at Home' which recognises that people with learning disabilities are constrained by the effects of abuse and neglect.

Physical disabilities

- *Working Together to Safeguard Children (HM Government 2006)* – has a specific section on the abuse of disabled children which highlights that disabled children may be especially vulnerable to abuse and guidance is given on handling concerns about and communicating with disabled children.
- *Youth and Criminal Justice Act (1999)* – defines vulnerable witnesses as all child witnesses under 17 years and any witness whose quality of evidence is likely to be diminished because they suffer from a mental disorder; have a significant impairment of intelligence and social functioning (learning disability); or have a physical disability or are suffering from a physical disorder.
- *Bullying involving Children with Special Educational Needs and Disabilities (DCSF 2008a)* – includes disabled children who are more at risk because of their impairment (i.e. may be less able to move away or may have cognitive impairments which make anticipation and avoidance difficult).

Black and ethnic minority issues

- *Delivering Race Equality in Mental Health Care (DH 2005a)* – sets out the Department of Health's policy on making mental health services more accessible to people from black and minority and ethnic backgrounds.
- *Female Genital Mutilation Act (2003)* – made it an offence for the first time for UK nationals or permanent UK residents to carry out FGM abroad, or to aid, abet, counsel or procure the carrying out of FGM abroad, even in countries in which the practice is legal, supported by guidance in *Working Together to Safeguard Children (HM Government 2006)*.
- *Dealing with cases of forced marriage – practice guidance for health professionals (FCO et al. 2007)* – aimed at police, social workers, education professionals and lawyers, to support the work of the government's Forced Marriage Unit jointly run by the Foreign and Commonwealth Office and Home Office.
- *Honour Based Violence* is included in *Working Together to Safeguard Children (HM Government 2006)* – as a collection of practices used to control behaviour within families to protect perceived cultural and religious beliefs about 'honour and perceived shame' dealt with by the family including physical violence and murder.

Appendix 2
Delphi questions

The questions were asked in relation to each of the 10 VVAPP programme areas; see Figure 1.1. Respondents answered for each area where they considered they had expertise by virtue of profession or experience.

Principles and core beliefs

1. What do you see as the most important principles and core beliefs to inform work with victims/survivors and/or perpetrators of sexual and domestic violence and abuse?

Effective interventions

2. If you are an academic or practitioner, what interventions work best in the support, care and treatment of victims/survivors and/or perpetrators?
    If you have expertise from personal experience, what treatments and interventions have worked best to help you live with and recover from your experience of sexual and domestic violence and abuse?
3. What practices or approaches should NOT be used and why?
4. If you are an academic or practitioner, which theoretical models and therapeutic approaches inform your work? If you have expertise from personal experience, what has helped you and why?
    Please mark relevant boxes. Please note you may mark more than one of these.
☐   PTSD/trauma therapy
☐   cognitive behavioural
☐   feminist/pro-feminist
☐   mediation/alternative dispute resolution
☐   family systems
☐   mutual support/self-help
☐   ecological/holistic
☐   art/drama therapy
☐   person-centred
☐   humanist

- ☐ psychodynamic/psychoanalysis
- ☐ recovery
- ☐ integrative theoretical model
- ☐ social learning theory
- ☐ restorative justice
- ☐ zero-tolerance
- ☐ relapse prevention
- ☐ group therapy
- ☐ other, please specify
  Please explain below the rationale for your preferred approach(es) and recommended psychological therapy(ies).

Managing safety and risk

5. What do those providing treatment, care and support need to know and do to ensure interventions are safe and effective for victims, survivors and abusers/perpetrators?

Training

6. What training and/or experience is required to provide effective interventions? What should this training involve and how should it be delivered?

Prevention

7. What needs to be done to prevent sexual and domestic violence and abuse?

Improving outcomes

8. What recommendations would you like to make to develop policy and practice to improve outcomes for individuals affected by sexual and domestic violence and abuse?

Addressing obstacles

9. What obstacles prevent these improvements and how can they be addressed?

The following options were offered for all questions:
DO NOT WISH TO ANSWER ☐
DO NOT KNOW THE ANSWER ☐
NOT APPLICABLE TO MY EXPERIENCE ☐

Appendix 3

Views on specific theoretical models and therapeutic approaches: percentage of Delphi experts who find particular approaches helpful, by programme area

Views on specific theoretical models and therapeutic approaches: percentage of Delphi experts who find particular approaches helpful, by programme area

| | Sexual violence | | | | | | Domestic violence and abuse | | | |
| | Victims/survivors | | | | Offenders | | Victims/survivors | | Perpetrators | |
	RSA adults %	CSA adults %	SA child & adol %	PPT %	IB/SA child & YP %	Adult %	Adult %	Child & adol %	Young people %	Adult %
Person-centred	56	58	48	53	29	27	52	45	27	22
PTSD/trauma therapy	43	51	48	42	39	24	38	43	27	24
Cognitive behavioural	37	45	40	47	52	61	29	33	27	54
Feminist/ pro-feminist	33	40	33	50	26	24	57	40	18	41
Group therapy	32	48	37	25	45	45	27	40	36	49
Psychodynamic/ psychoanalysis	37	44	37	42	35	27	28	33	45	32
Mutual support/ self-help	34	37	35	39	13	18	42	50	18	30
Art/drama therapy	32	35	45	39	35	27	24	48	36	22
Family systems	30	29	43	31	52	33	20	35	45	41
Humanist	33	37	22	25	13	9	27	20	18	16

Views on specific theoretical models and therapeutic approaches: percentage of Delphi experts who find particular approaches helpful, by programme area – continued

Integrative theoretical model	28	35	25	25	13	33	18	18	9	24
Ecological/holistic	17	24	20	28	26	12	16	23	27	16
Recovery	15	22	18	19	13	6	15	18	9	11
Relapse prevention	10	13	12	17	32	36	8	10	0	30
Social learning theory	8	7	7	11	26	30	13	10	18	27
Zero-tolerance	9	8	8	8	0	9	17	18	36	22
Mediation/ alternative dispute resolution	5	6	3	17	3	6	6	8	18	8
Restorative justice	7	5	2	6	6	6	2	5	9	8
Number of respondents	99	123	60	36	31	33	99	40	11	37

Key: CSA childhood sexual abuse, IB/SA sexually inappropriate behaviour/sexually abuse, PPT prostitution, pornography and trafficking, RSA rape and sexual assault, YP young people.

Source: responses from Q4, Round 1 of Delphi consultation.

References

Abel, G.G., Mittelman, M.S., and Becker, J.V. (1985) 'Sexual offenders: Results of assessment and recommendations for treatment', in M.H. Ben-Aron, S.J. Hucker, and C.D. Webster (eds), *Clinical criminology: The assessment and treatment of criminal behaviour*, Toronto: M&G Graphic.

Abrahams, C. (1994) *The hidden victims: Children and domestic violence*, London: NCH Action for Children.

Adi, Y., Ashcroft, D., Browne, K., Beech, A., Fry-Smith, A. and Hyde, C. (2002) 'Clinical effectiveness and cost-consequences of selective serotonin reuptake inhibitors in the treatment of sex offenders', *Health Technology Assessment*, 6(28).

Akuffo, E.O. and Sylvester, P.E. (1983) 'Head injury and mental handicap', *Journal of the Royal Society of Medicine*, 76: 545–9.

Alarid, L. (2000) 'Sexual assault and coercion among incarcerated women prisoners: Excerpts from prison letters', *Prison Journal*, 80(4): 391–406.

Ammerman, R.T., Van Hasselt, V.B. and Hersen, M. (1988) 'Maltreatment of handicapped children: A critical review', *Journal of Family Violence*, 3(1): 53–72.

Anderson, T.R. and Aviles, A.M. (2006) 'Diverse faces of domestic violence', *ABNF Journal*, 17(4): 129–32.

Antecol, H. and Cobb-Clark, D. (2001) 'Men, women, and sexual harassment in the U.S. military', *Gender Issues*, 19(1): 3–18.

Arata, C. (2002) 'Child sexual abuse and sexual revictimization', *Clinical Psychology: Science and Practice*, 9(2): 135–64.

Archer, J. (2000) 'Sex differences in aggression between heterosexual partners: A meta-analytic review', *Psychological Bulletin*, 126 (5): 651–80.

Archer, J. (2002) 'Sex differences in physically aggressive acts between heterosexual partners: A meta-analytic review', *Aggression and Violent Behavior*, 7: 313–51.

Arriola, K.R.J., Louden, T., Doldren, M.A. and Fortenberry, R.M. (2005) 'A meta-analysis of the relationship of child sexual abuse to HIV risk behavior among women', *Child Abuse and Neglect*, 29: 725–46.

Babcock, J.C., Green, C.E. and Robie, C. (2004) 'Does batterers' treatment work? A meta-analytic review of domestic violence treatment', *Clinical Psychology Review*, 23: 1023–53.

Bacon. H., and Richardson, S. (2000) 'Child sexual abuse and the continuum of victim disclosure: Professionals working with children in Cleveland in 1987', in C. Itzin (ed.), *Home truths about child sexual abuse: Influencing policy and practice*, London: Routledge.

BACP (2006) *Ethical framework for good practice in counselling and psychother-apy: Ethics for counselling and psychotherapy*. Online. Available <http://www.bacp.co.uk/ethical_framework/> (accessed 17 June 2006).

Bailey, S. (2000) 'Sadistic, sexual and violent acts in the young: Contributing factors', in C. Itzin (ed.), *Home truths about child sexual abuse: Influencing policy and practice*, London: Routledge.

Bair-Merritt, M.H., Blackstone, M. and Feudtner, C. (2006) 'Physical health out-comes of childhood exposure to intimate partner violence: a systematic review', *Pediatrics*, 117(2): 278–90.

Barile, M. (2002) 'Individual-systemic violence: Disabled women's standpoint', *Journal of International Women's Studies*, 4(1): 1–14.

Barron, P., Hassiotis, A. and Barnes, J. (2002) 'Offenders with intellectual disability: The size of the problem and therapeutic outcomes', *Journal of Intellectual Disability Research*, 46(6): 454–63.

Beaulaurier, R.L., Seff, L.R., Newman, F.L. and Dunlop, B. (2007) 'External barri-ers to help seeking for older women who experience intimate partner violence', *Journal of Family Violence*, 22: 747–55.

Bentovim, A., Cox, A., Miller, L.B. and Pizzey, S. (2009) *Safeguarding children living with trauma and violence*, London: Jessica Kingsley Publishers.

Bicknell, J. (1983) 'The psychopathology of handicap', *British Journal of Medical Psychology*, 56: 167–78.

Biering, P. (2007) 'Adapting the concept of explanatory models of illness to the study of youth violence', *Journal of Interpersonal Violence*, 22(7): 791–811.

Birrell, R. and Birrell, J. (1968) 'The maltreatment syndrome in children: A hospital survey', *Medical Journal of Australia*, 2: 1023–29.

Blackman, N. (2003) *Loss and learning disability*, London: Worth.

Blinn-Pike, L., Berger, T., Dixon, D., Kuschel, D. and Kaplan, M. (2002) 'Is there a causal link between maltreatment and adolescent pregnancy? A literature review', *Perspectives on Sexual and Reproductive Health*, 34(2): 68–75.

Bone, M. and Meltzer, H. (1989) *The prevalence of disability among children, OPCS surveys of disability in Great Britain Report 3*, London: HMSO.

Bonomi, A.E., Thompson, R.S., Anderson, M., Reid R.J., Carrell, D., Dimer, J.A. and Rivara, F.P. (2006) 'Intimate partner violence and women's physical, mental, and social functioning', *American Journal of Preventive Medicine*, 30(6): 458–66.

Booth, B. and Grogan, M. (1990) *People with learning difficulties who sexually offend*, Ashton-under-Lyne: Community Resource Centre, Tameside General Hospital.

Bornstein, R.F. (2005) 'Interpersonal dependency in child abuse perpetrators and victims: A meta-analytic review', *Journal of Psychopathology and Behavioral Assessment*, 27(2): 67–76.

Bostock, J., Plumpton, M. and Pratt, R. (2009) 'Domestic violence against women: Understanding social processes and women's experiences', *Journal of Community and Applied Social Psychology*, 19(2): 95–110.

Boy, A. and Salihu, H.M. (2004) 'Intimate partner violence and birth outcomes: A systematic review', *International Journal of Fertility*, 49(4): 159–63.

Brandon, M., Bailey, S., Belderson, P., Gardner R., Sidebotham, P., Dodsworth, J., Warren, C. and Black, J. (2009) *Understanding Serious Case Reviews and their Impact: A biennial analysis of serious case reviews 2005–07*, London: DCSF Research report DCSF – RR129.

Brandon, M., Belderson, P., Warren, C., Howe, D., Gardner, R., Dodsworth, J. and Black, J. (2008) *Analysing child deaths and serious injury through abuse and neglect: What can we learn? A biennial analysis of serious case reviews 2003–2005*, London: DCSF Research report DCSF – RR023.

Breen, T. and Turk, V. (1991) 'Sexual offending behaviour by people with learning disabilities, prevalence and treatment', Unpublished Paper, Canterbury: University of Kent.

Briere, J. and Jordan, C.E. (2009) 'Childhood maltreatment, intervening variables and adult psychological difficulties in women', *Trauma, Violence and Abuse*, 10(4): 375–88.

Briken, P., Hill, A. and Berner, W. (2003) 'Pharmacotherapy of paraphilias with long-acting agonists if luteinizing hormone-releasing hormone: A systematic review', *Journal of Clinical Psychiatry*, 64(8): 890–7.

British Council (1999) *Violence against women: A briefing document on international issues and responses*, Manchester: The British Council.

Bruder, C. and Stenfert Kroese, B. (2005) 'The efficacy of interventions designed to prevent and protect people with intellectual disabilities from sexual abuse: A review of the literature', *The Journal of Adult Protection*, 7(2): 13–27.

Bryant-Davis, T., Chung, H. and Tillman, S. (2009) 'From the margins to the center: Ethnic minority women and the mental health effects of sexual assault', *Trauma, Violence and Abuse*, 10(4): 330–57.

Buchanan, A. and Oliver, J.E. (1979) 'Abuse and neglect as a cause of mental retardation', *Child Abuse and Neglect*, 3: 467–75.

Buchbinder, E. and Eisikovits, Z. (2008) 'Doing treatment: Batterers' experience of intervention', *Children and Youth Services Review*, 30: 616–30.

Bunting, L. (2005) *Females who sexually offend against children: Responses of the child protection and criminal justice systems*, London: NSPCC.

Burris, C.T. and Jackson, L.M. (1999) 'Hate the sin/love the sinner, or love the hater? Intrinsic religion and responses to partner abuse', *Journal for the Scientific Study of Religion*, 38(1): 160–74.

Butler, S.M. and Seto, M.C. (2002) 'Distinguishing two types of adolescent sex offenders', *Journal of the American Academy of Child and Adolescent Psychiatry*, 41: 83–90.

Buzawa, E.S. and Buzawa, C.G. (2003) *Domestic violence: The criminal justice response*, London: Sage.

Campbell, D. (1989) 'A psychoanalytic contribution to understanding delinquents at school', *Journal of Educational Therapy*, 2(4): 50–65.

Campbell, J.C. (2002) 'Health consequences of intimate partner violence', *Lancet*, 359: 1331–6.

Carlson, B.E. (2000) 'Children exposed to intimate partner violence: Research findings and implications for intervention', *Trauma, Violence and Abuse*, 1(4): 321–42.

Cartor, P., Cimbolic, P. and Tallon, J. (2008) 'Differentiating pedophilia from ephebophilia in cleric offenders', *Sexual Addition and Compulsivity*, 15(4): 311–19.

Cawson, P. (2002) *Child Maltreatment in the Family: – The experience of a national sample of young people*, London: NSPCC.

Cawson, Wattam, C., Brooker, S. and Kelly, G. (2000) *Child maltreatment in the UK: A study of prevalence of child abuse and neglect*, London: NSPCC.

Chase, E. and Statham, J. (2005) 'Commercial and sexual exploitation of children and young people in the UK: A review', *Child Abuse Review*, 14: 4–25.

Chenoweth, L. (1997) 'Violence and women with disabilities: silence and paradox', in S. Cook and J. Bessant (eds), *Women's encounters with violence: Australian experiences*, Thousand Oaks, CA: Sage.

Chibnall, J.T., Wolf, A. and Duckro, P.N. (1998) 'A national survey of the sexual trauma experiences of Catholic nuns', *Review of Religious Research*, 40(2): 142–67.

Choi, H., Klein, C., Shin, M.-S. and Lee, H.-J. (2009) 'Posttraumatic Stress Disorder (PTSD) and Disorders of Extreme Stress (DESNOS) symptoms following prostitution and childhood abuse', *Violence Against Women*, 15(8): 933–51.

Cicchetti, D. and Rogosch, F.A. (1997) 'The role of self-organization in the promotion of resilience in maltreated children', *Development and Psychopathology*, 9: 797–815.

Classen, C.C., Gronskaya Palesh, O. and Aggarwal, R. (2005) 'Sexual revictimisation: A review of the empirical literature', *Trauma, Violence and Abuse*, 6(2): 103–29.

Cohen, J.A., Mannarino, A.P., Murray, L.K. and Igelman, R. (2006) 'Psychosocial interventions for maltreated and violence-exposed children', *Journal of Social Issues*, 62(4): 737–66.

Cohen, S. and Warren, R. (1987) 'Preliminary survey of family abuse of children served by united cerebral palsy centers', *Developmental Medicine and Child Neurology*, 29: 12–18.

Cole, M., Baldwin, D. and Thomas, P. (2003) 'Sexual assault on wards: Staff actions and reactions', *International Journal of Psychiatry in Clinical Practice*, 7(4): 239–42.

Coleman, K., Jansson, K., Kaiza, P. and Reed, R. (2007) *Homicides, firearm offences and intimate violence 2005/2006* (Supplementary Volume 1 to Crime in England and Wales 2005/2006), London: Home Office.

Collin-Vezina, D. and Hebert, M. (2005) 'Comparing dissociation and PTSD in sexually abused school-aged girls', *Journal of Nervous and Mental Disease*, 193: 47–52.

Commission to Inquire into Child Abuse (2009) *The Ryan Report*, Available at: <http://www.childabusecommission.com/rpt/04-06.php>.

Connell R.W. (1987) *Gender and power: Society, the person and sexual politics*, Cambridge: Polity Press.

Cooke, L.B. (1990) 'Abuse of mentally handicapped adults', *Psychiatric Bulletin*, 14: 608–9.

Cooke, P. and Standen, P.J. (2002) 'Abuse and disabled children: Hidden needs?' *Child Abuse Review*, 11: 1–18.

Cooper, C., Selwood, A. and Livingston, G. (2008) 'The prevalence of elder abuse and neglect: A systematic review', *Age and Ageing*, 37(2): 151–60.

Copel, L.C. (2008) 'The lived experience of women in abusive relationships who sought spiritual guidance', *Issues in Mental Health Nursing*, 29: 115–30.

Corcoran, J. and Pillai, V. (2008) 'A meta-analysis of parent-involved treatment for child sexual abuse', *Research on Social Work Practice*, 18(5): 453–64.

Cottis, T. (2009) *Intellectual disability, trauma and disability*, London: Routledge.

Coulthard, P., Yong, S.L., Adamson, L., Warburton, A., Worthington, H.V. and Esposito, M. (2004) 'Domestic violence screening and intervention programmes for adults with dental or facial injury (Review)', *Cochrane Database of Systematic Reviews*, 2004(2).

Courtney, J. and Rose, J. (2004) 'The effectiveness of treatment for male sex offenders with learning disabilities: A review of the literature', *Journal of Sexual Aggression*, 10(2): 215–36.

CPS (2001) *Provision of therapy for child witnesses prior to a criminal trial: Practice guidance*. Online. Available HTTP: <http://www.cps.gov.uk/publications/prosecution/therapychild.html> (accessed 3 March 2010).

Cross, M. (1999) *Proud child, Safer child*, London: Women's Press.

Curen, R. (2009) 'Can they see in the door: Assessment and treatment of learning disabled sex offenders', in T. Cottis (ed.), *Intellectual disability, trauma and disability*, London: Routledge.

Davenport, R., Hester, M., Regan, L. and Williamson, E. (forthcoming) *Exploring the service and support needs of male, lesbian, gay, bi-sexual and transgendered and black and other minority ethnic victims of sexual violence: Rapid Evidence Assessment (REA) of the literature*, London: Home Office.

Davis, L.A. (2000) 'More common than we think: Recognizing and responding to signs of violence', *Impact,* 13(3). Online. Available at: <http://ici.umn.edu/products/impact/133/default.html> (accessed 5 November 2009).

DCSF (2007a) *Safeguarding children from sexual exploitation*, London: DCSF.

DCSF (2007b) *Safeguarding children who may have been trafficked*, London: DCSF.

DCSF (2008a) *Bullying involving children with special educational needs and disabilities. Safe to learn: Embedding anti-bullying work in schools*, London: DCSF.

DCSF (2008b) *Staying safe: Action plan*, London: DCSF.

De Coster, S., Estes, S.B. and Mueller., C.W. (1999) 'Routine activities and sexual harassment in the workplace', *Work and Occupations* 26: 21–49.

DeLeon-Granados,W. and Long, J. (2000) 'The case of the tree that battered a woman: An analysis of the language of domestic violence calls for service', paper presented at the annual meeting of the American Society of Criminology, San Francisco, CA, November, 2000.

DeLeon-Granados, W., Wells, W. and Binsbacher, R. (2006) 'Arresting developments, trends in female arrests for domestic violence and proposed explanations', *Violence Against Women*, 12 (4): 355–71.

Department of Defense (2004) *Taguba Report*. Online. Available HTTP: <http://www.dod.mil/pubs/foi/detainees/taguba/TAGUBA_REPORT_CERTIFICATIONS.pdf> (accessed 9 November 2009).

Depoy, E., Gilson, S. and Cramer, E. (2003) 'Understanding the experiences of and advocating for the service and resource needs of abused, disabled women', in A. Hans and A. Pat (eds), *Women, disability and identity*, London: Sage.

DES (2006a) *Children in Need in England: Results of a survey of activity and expenditure as reported by Local Authority Social Services Children and Families Teams for a survey week in February 2005: National Statistics, Communities*, Bristol: The Policy Press.

DES (2006b) *Bullying around racism, religion and culture*, London: DES.

DH (1999) *Mental health national service framework*, London: DH.

DH (2001) *Valuing people with learning disabilities A new strategy for learning disability for the 21st century*, London: Stationery Office.

DH (2002a) *National suicide prevention strategy for England*, London: DH.

DH (2002b) *Women's mental health: Into the mainstream. Strategic development of mental health care of women*, London: DH.

DH (2003) *Mainstreaming gender and women's mental health*, London: DH.

DH (2004a) *Protection of vulnerable adults scheme in England and Wales for care homes and domiciliary care agencies: A practical guide*, London: DH.

DH (2004b) *Choosing health: Making healthy choices easier*, London: DH.

DH (2005a) *Delivering race equality in mental health care*, London: DH.

DH (2005b) *Responding to domestic abuse: A handbook for health professionals*, London: DH.

DH (2005c) *Delivering choosing health: Making healthy choices easier*, London: DH.

DH (2008) *Healthier, fairer and safer communities: Towards a framework for violence and abuse prevention*, London: DH.

DH and DES (2004) *National service framework for children, young people and maternity*, London: DH/DES.

DH and HO (2000) *No secrets: Guidance on developing and implementing multi-agency policies and procedures to protect vulnerable adults from abuse*, London: DH.

DH and HO (2006) *Domestic abuse training manual for health professionals*, London: DH and HO. Online. Available HTTP: <http://www.crimereduction. homeoffice.gov.uk/domesticviolence/domesticviolence58.htm> (accessed 21 February 2010).

DH, HO and ACPO (2009) *A resource for developing sexual assault referral centres (SARCs)*, London: DH, HO and ACPO.

Diamond, L.J. and Jaudes, P.K. (1983) 'Child abuse in a cerebral palsied population', *Developmental Medicine and Child Neurology*, 25 (2): 169–74.

Disch, E. and Avery, N. (2001) 'Sex in the consulting room, the examining room, and the sacristy: Survivors of sexual abuse by professionals', *American Journal of Orthopsychiatry*, 71(2): 204–17.

Dixon, M., Reed, H., Rogers, B. and Stone, L. (2006) *Crime share: The unequal impact of crime*, London: Institute for Public Policy Research.

Dobash, R.P. and Dobash, R.E. (2003) 'Violence in intimate relationships', in W. Heitmeyer and J. Hagan (eds), *International handbook of violence research*, Dordrecht: Kluwer Academic Publishers.

Dobash, R.P. and Dobash, R.E. (2004) 'Women's violence to men in intimate relationships', *British Journal of Criminology*, 44: 324–49.

Dobson, B. and Middleton, S. (1998) *Paying to care: The cost of childhood disability*, York: YPS.

Dodd, T. Nicholas, S., Povey, D. and Walker, A. (2004) *Crime in England and Wales 2003/4*, London: Office of National Statistics.

Donovan, C. and Hester, M. (2007) *Comparing love and domestic violence in heterosexual and same sex relationships: Full research report*, ESRC End of Award Report, RES-000-23-0650, Swindon: ESRC.

Donovan, C. and Hester, M. (2008) ' "Because she was my first girlfriend, I didn't know any different": Making the case for mainstreaming same-sex sex/ relationship education', *Sex Education*, 8(3): 277–88.

Dowden, C., Antonowicz, D. and Andrews, D.A. (2003) 'The effectiveness of relapse prevention with offenders: A meta-analysis', *International Journal of Offender Therapy and Comparative Criminology*, 47(5): 516–28.

Downs, W.R., Rindels, B. and Atkinson, C. (2007) 'Women's use of physical and nonphysical self-defense strategies during incidents of partner violence', *Violence Against Women*, 13 (1): 28–45.

Doyle, T.P. (2006) 'Clericalism: Enabler of clergy sexual abuse', *Pastoral Psychology*, 54(3): 189–213.

DRC (2006) *Ending child poverty: the disability dimension*, London: Disability Rights Commission.

Dubowitz, H., Feigelman, S., Lane, W. and Kim, J. (2009) 'Pediatric primary care to help prevent child maltreatment: The Safe Environment for Every Kid (SEEK) model', *Pediatrics*, 123(3): 858–64.

Dumond, R. (2000) 'Inmate sexual assault: The plague that persists', *Prison Journal*, 80(4): 407–14.

Dyson, C. (2008) *Poverty and child maltreatment Research Briefing*, London: NSPCC.

Eckhardt, C.I., Murphy, C., Black, D. and Suhr, L. (2006) 'Intervention programs for perpetrators of intimate partner violence: Conclusions from a clinical research perspective', *Public Health Reports*, 121(4): 369–81.

EDCM (2007) *Disabled children and child poverty*, Briefing Paper by the Every Disabled Child Matters campaign, London: EDCM. Online. Available: <http://www.edcm.org.uk/pdfs/disabled_children_and_child_poverty.pdf> (accessed 5 November 2009).

Edleson, J. (1999a) 'Children's witnessing of adult domestic violence', *Journal of Interpersonal Violence*, 14(8): 839–70.

Edleson, J. (1999b) 'The overlap between child maltreatment and woman battering', *Violence Against Women*, 5(2): 134–54.

Equality and Human Rights Commission (2006) *Gender equality duty*. Online. Available HTTP: <http://www.equalityhumanrights.com/advice-and-guidance/public-sector-duties/what-are-the-public-sector-duties/gender-equality-duty/> (accessed 3 March 2010).

Equality and Human Rights Commission (2008) *Single equality duty*. Online. Available HTTP: <http://www.equalityhumanrights.com/advice-and-guidance/public-sector-duties/what-are-the-public-sector-duties/single-equality-duty/> (accessed 3 March 2010).

Eriksson, M., Hester, M., Keskinen, S. and Pringle, K. (eds) (2005) *Tackling men's violence in families: Nordic issues and dilemmas*, Bristol: Policy Press.

Evans, E., Hawton, K. and Rodham, K. (2004) 'Factors associated with suicidal phenomena in adolescents: A systematic review of population-based studies', *Clinical Psychology Review*, 24 (8): 957–79.

Evans, E., Hawton, K. and Rodham, K. (2005) 'Suicidal phenomena and abuse in adolescents: A review of epidemiological studies', *Child Abuse and Neglect*, 29(1): 45–58.

Evans, S.E., Davies, C. and DiLillo, D. (2008) 'Exposure to domestic violence: A meta-analysis of child and adolescent outcomes', *Aggression and Violent Behavior*, 13(2): 131–40.

Fargo, J.D. (2008) 'Pathways to adult sexual revictimization: Direct and indirect behavioural risk factors across the lifespan', *Journal of Interpersonal Violence*, 24(11): 1771–91.

Farmer, E.R.G. and Owen, M. (1995) *Child protection practice: Private risks and public remedies*, London: HMSO.

Farmer, E.R.G. and Owen, M. (2000) 'Gender and the child protection process', in J. Hanmer and C. Itzin (eds), *Home truths about child sexual abuse: Influencing policy and practice*, London: Routledge.

FCO, HO and NHS (2007) *Dealing with cases of forced marriage: Practice guidance for health professionals*, London: FCO, HO and NHS.

Fear, N.T. and Williamson, S. (2003) *Suicide and open verdict deaths among males in the UK regular armed forces: Comparison with the UK civilian population and the US military*, London: Defence Analytic Services Agency.

Feder, G.S., Hutson, M., Ramsay, J. and Taket, A.R. (2006) 'Expectations and experiences of women experiencing intimate partner violence when they encounter health care professionals: A meta-analysis of qualitative studies', *Archives of Internal Medicine*, 166: 22–37.

Feder, G., Ramsay, J., Dunne, D., Rose, M., Arsene, C., Norman, R., Kuntze, S., Spencer, A., Bacchus, L., Hague, G., Warburton, A. and Taket, A. (2009) 'How far does screening women for domestic (partner) violence in different health care settings meet criteria for a screening programme? Systematic reviews of nine UK National Screening Committee criteria', *Health Technology Assessment*, 13(16): 1–113. Available at <http://www.hta.ac.uk/fullmono/mon1316.pdf> (accessed 5 November 2009).

Feder, L. and Wilson, D.B. (2005) 'A meta-analytic review of court-mandated batterer intervention programs: Can courts affect abusers' behavior?' *Journal of Experimental Criminology*, 2005(1): 239–62.

Field, C.A. and Caetano, R. (2004) 'Ethnic differences in intimate partner violence in the U.S. general population: The role of alcohol use and socioeconomic status', *Trauma, Violence and Abuse*, 5(4): 303–17.

Finkelhor, D. (1994) 'The international epidemiology of child sexual abuse', *Child Abuse and Neglect*, 18(5): 409–17.

Finney, A. (2006) *Domestic violence, sexual assault and stalking: findings from the 2004/05 British Crime Survey*, Home Office Online Report 12/06. Online. Available HHTP: <http:// http://rds.homeoffice.gov.uk/rds/pdfs06/rdsolr1206.pdf> (accessed 25 May 2010).

Fouque, P. and Glachan, M. (2000) 'The impact of Christian counselling on survivors of sexual abuse', *Counselling Psychology Quarterly*, 13(2): 201–20.

Frank, K. (2003) ' "Just Trying to Relax": Masculinity, masculinizing practices, and strip club regulars', *The Journal of Sex Research*, 40(1): 61–75.

Frodi, A.M. (1981) 'Contributions of infant characteristics to child abuse', *American Journal of Mental Deficiency*, 85(4): 341–9.

Gabe, J. and Elston, M.A. (2008) "We don't have to take this': Zero tolerance of violence against health care workers in a time of insecurity', *Social Policy and Administration*, 42(6): 691–709.

Gallagher, B., Bradford, M. and Pease, K. (2008) 'Attempted and completed incidents of stranger-perpetrated child sexual abuse and abduction', *Child Abuse and Neglect*, 32(5): 517–28.

Garcia-Moreno, C. and Watts, C. (2000) 'Violence against women: Its importance for HIV and AIDS', *AIDS*, 14(suppl): S253–S265.

Garcia-Moreno, C., Jansen, H., Ellsberg, M., Heise, L. and Watts, C. (2006) 'Prevalence of intimate partner violence: Findings from the WHO multi-country study on women's health and domestic violence', *Lancet*, 368: 1260–9.

Garfield, S. (2007) 'Exploring the impact of the therapeutic alliance and structural factors in treatment groups for domestically abusive men', Unpublished Ph.D. thesis, London: London South Bank University.

Gazmararian, J.A., Petersen, R., Spitz, A.M., Goodwin, M.M., Saltzman, L.E. and Marks, J.S. (2000) 'Violence and reproductive health: Current knowledge and future research directions', *Maternal and Child Health Journal*, 4(2): 79–84.

Gilby, R., Wolf, L. and Goldberg, B. (1989) 'Mentally retarded adolescent sex offenders: A survey and pilot study', *Canadian Journal of Psychiatry*, 34: 542–8.

Glaser, D. (2000) 'Child abuse and neglect and the brain: A review', *Journal of Child Psychology*, 41(1): 97–116.

Glasser, M. (1996) 'Aggression and sadism in the perversions', in I. Rosen (ed.), *Sexual deviation* (3rd edn), Oxford: Oxford University Press.

Glick, P., Sakalli-Ugurlu, N., Ferreira, M.C. and de Souza, M.A. (2002) 'Ambivalent sexism and attitudes toward wife abuse in Turkey and Brazil', *Psychology of Women Quarterly*, 26(4): 292–7.

Godenzi, A. and Yodanis, C. (1998) *Erster Bericht zu den ökonomischen Kosten der Gewalt gegen Frauen (First report of the economic expense of violence against women)*, Freiburg: University of Freiburg.

Godsi, E. (2004) *Violence and Society: Making sense of madness and badness*, Ross on Wye: PCCS Books.

Golding, J. (1999) 'Intimate partner violence as a risk factor for mental disorders: A meta-analysis', *Journal of Family Violence*, 14(2): 99–132.

Gonzalez, A. and MacMillan H. L. (2008) 'Preventing child maltreatment: An evidence-based update', *Journal of Postgraduate Medicine* 54(4): 280–6.

Goodman, L.A., Fels Smyth, K., Borges, A.M. and Singer, R. (2009) 'When crises collide: How intimate partner violence and poverty intersect to shape women's mental health and coping', *Trauma, Violence and Abuse*, 10(4): 306–29.

Gordon, D., Townsend, P., Levitas, R., Pantazis, C., Payne, S., Patsios, D., Middleton, S., Ashworth, K., Adelman, L., Bradshaw, J., Williams, J. and Bramley, G. (2000) *Poverty and social exclusion in Britain*, York: Joseph Rowntree Foundation.

Griffiths, D., Hingsburger, D. and Christian, R. (1985) 'Treating developmentally handicapped sexual offenders: The York behaviour management services treatment program', *Psychiatric Aspects in Mental Retardation Reviews*, 4: 49–52.

Hackett, S. (2004) *What works for children and young people with harmful sexual behaviours?* Barkingside: Barnardo's.

Hagemann-White, C. (2001) 'European research on the prevalence of violence against women', *Violence Against Women*, 7(7): 732–59.

Hague, G., Thiara, R., Magowan, P. and Mullender, A. (2008a) *Making the links: Disabled women and domestic violence, Final Report*, Bristol: Women's Aid.

Hague, G., Thiara, R., Magowan, P. and Mullender, A. (2008b) *Making the links: Disabled women and domestic violence, Summary of findings and recommendations for good practice*, Bristol: Women's Aid.

Hahn, R.A., Bilukha, O.O., Crosby, A., Fullilove, M., Liberman, A., Moscicki, E., Snyder, S., Tuma, F., Schofield, A., Corso, P. and Briss, P. (2003) 'First reports evaluating the effectiveness of strategies for preventing violence: early childhood home visitation: Findings from the Task Force on Community Preventive Services', *Morbidity and Mortality Weekly Report Recommendations and Reports*, 52(14): 1–9.

Haj-Yahia, M.M. (2002) 'Beliefs of Jordanian women about wife-beating', *Psychology of Women Quarterly*, 26(4): 282–91.

Hamberger, L.K. and Guse, C.E. (2002) 'Men's and women's use of intimate partner violence in clinical samples', *Violence Against Women*, 8: 1301–31.

Hanmer, J. (2000) 'Domestic violence and gender relations: contexts and connections', in J. Hanmer and C. Itzin (eds), *Home truths about domestic violence: Feminist influences on policy and practice: A reader*, London: Routledge.

Hanson, R.K. and Morton-Bourgon, K.E. (2005) 'The characteristics of persistent sexual offenders: A meta-analysis of recidivism studies', *Journal of Consulting and Clinical Psychology*, 73(6): 1154–63.

Hanson, R.K., Gordon, A., Harris, A.J.R., Marques, J.K., Murphy, W., Quinsey, V.L. and Seto, M.C. (2002) 'First report of the collaborative outcome data project on the effectiveness of psychological treatment for sex offenders', *Sex Abuse*, 14(2): 169–94.

Haque, S. (2009) 'Differences, differences, differences: Working with ethnic cultural and religious diversity', in T. Cottis (ed.), *Intellectual disability, trauma and disability*, London: Routledge.

Hard, S. and Plumb, W. (1987) 'Sexual abuse of persons with developmental disabilities: A case study', Unpublished manuscript annotated in H. Brown and V. Turk (eds) *Sexual abuse and people with learning difficulties Annotated Bibliography*, 1991, Canterbury: University of Kent, Centre for Applied Psychology of Social Care.

Harper, K., Stalker, C.A., Palmer, S. and Gadbois, S. (2008) 'Adults traumatized by child abuse: What survivors need from community-based mental health professionals', *Journal of Mental Health*, 17(4): 361–74.

Hartling, L.M. (2008) 'Strengthening resilience in a risky world: It's all about relationships', *Women and Therapy*, 31(2-4): 51–70.

Hartman, J.L., Turner, M.G., Daigle, L.E., Exum, M.L. and Cukken, F.T. (2009) 'Exploring the gender differences in protective factors: Implications for understanding resiliency', *International Journal of Offender Therapy and Comparative Criminology*, 53(3): 249–77.

Hass, M. and Graydon, K. (2009) 'Sources of resiliency among successful foster youth', *Children and Youth Services Review*, 31: 457–63.

Hathaway, J.E., Zimmer, B., Willis, G. and Silverman, J.G. (2008) 'Perceived changes in health and safety following participation in a health care-based domestic violence program', *Journal of Midwifery and Women's Health*, 53(6): 547–55.

Havig, K. (2008) 'The health care experiences of adult survivors of child sexual abuse: A systematic review of evidence on sensitive practice', *Trauma Violence and Abuse*, 9(1): 19–33.

Hearn, J. (1996) 'Men's violence to known women: Historical, everyday and theoretical constructions by men', in B. Fawcett, B. Featherstone, J. Hearn and C. Toft (eds), *Violence and Gender Relations*, London: Sage.

Hedin, L.W. (2000) 'Physical and sexual abuse against women and children', *Current Opinion in Obstetrics and Gynecology*, 12(5): 349–55.

Heise, L.L. (1998) 'Violence against women: An integrated, ecological framework', *Violence Against Women*, 4: 262–90.

Heise, L.L., Ellsberg, M. and Gottemoeller, M. (1999) *Ending violence against women*, Baltimore, MD: Johns Hopkins University School of Public Health, Center for Communications Programs (Population Reports, Series L, No. 11).

Heiskanen, M. and Piispa, M. (2001) *The price of violence. The costs of men's violence against women in Finland*, Helsinki: Statistics Finland.

Herrenkohl, E.C., Herrenkohl, R.C. and Egolf, B.P. (1983) 'Circumstances surrounding the occurrence of child maltreatment', *Journal of Consulting and Clinical Psychology*, 51: 424–31.

Herrington, V., Harvey, S., Hunter, G. and Hough, M., (2007) *Assessing the prevalence of learning disability among young adult offenders in Feltham*, London: Institute for Criminal Policy Research School of Law Publication, King's College London.

Herspring, D. (2005) 'Dedovshchina in the Russian army: The problem that won't go away', *Journal of Slavic Military Studies*, 18(4): 607–29.

Herzog, S. (2004) 'Differential perceptions of the seriousness of male violence against female intimate partners among Jews and Arabs in Israel', *Journal of Interpersonal Violence*, 19(8): 891–900.

Hester, M. (1992) *Lewd women and wicked witches: A study of the dynamics of male domination*, London: Routledge.

Hester, M. (2004) 'Future trends and developments: Violence against women in Europe and East Asia', *Violence Against Women*, 10 (12): 1431–48.

Hester, M. (2006) 'Making it through the criminal justice system: Attrition and domestic violence', *Social Policy and Society*, 5 (1): 79–90.

Hester, M. (2009) *Who does what to whom? Gender and domestic violence perpetrators*, Bristol: University of Bristol in association with Northern Rock Foundation.

Hester, M. and Donovan, C. (2009) Researching domestic violence in same sex relationships: A feminist epistemological approach to survey development', *Lesbian Studies*, 13(2): 161–73.

Hester, M. and Westmarland, N. (2005) *Tackling domestic violence: Effective interventions and approaches*, Home Office Research Study 290, London: Home Office.

Hester, M. and Westmarland, N. (2007) 'Domestic violence perpetrators', *Criminal Justice Matters*, 66: 34–6.

Hester, M., Pearson, C. and Harwin, N. (2007) *Making an impact:– Children and domestic violence: a reader* (2nd edn), London, Philadelphia: Jessica Kingsley Publishers.

Hester, M., Westmarland, N., Gangoli, G., Wilkinson, M., O'Kelly, C., Kent, A. and Diamond, A. (2006) *Domestic violence perpetrators: Identifying needs to inform early intervention*, Bristol: University of Bristol in association with the Northern Rock Foundation and the Home Office.

Hester, M., Donovan, C. and Fahmy, E. (2010) 'Feminist epistemology and the politics of method: Surveying same sex domestic violence', *International Journal of Social Research Methodology*, 13(3): 251-63.

Hester, M., Regan, L. and Williamson, E., Davenport, R., Gangoli, G., Coulter, M., Chantler, K. and Green, L. (forthcoming) *Exploring the service and support needs of male, lesbian, gay, bi-sexual and transgendered and black and other minority ethnic victims of domestic and sexual violence*, London: Home Office.

Hetzel-Riggin, M.D., Brausch, A.M. and Montgomery, B.S. (2007) 'A meta-analytic investigation of therapy modality outcomes for sexually abused children and adolescents: an exploratory study', *Child Abuse and Neglect*, 31: 125–41.

Hickman, L.J., Jaycox, L.H. and Aronoff, J. (2004) 'Dating violence among adolescents: Prevalence, gender distribution and prevention program effectiveness', *Trauma, Violence and Abuse*, 5(2): 123–42.

HM Government (2006) *Working together to safeguard children: A guide to interagency working to safeguard and promote the welfare of children*, London: Stationery Office.

HM Government (2007) *Cross government action plan on sexual violence and abuse*, London: Stationery Office.

HM Government (2009) *Valuing People Now: A new three year strategy for people with learning disabilities – making it happen for everyone*, London: DH.

HM Treasury (2004) *Child poverty review*, London: Stationery Office.

HM Treasury and DES (2007) *Policy review of children and young people: A discussion paper*, London: Stationery Office.

HO (2005a) 'Domestic violence delivery plan', Annex A in *Domestic violence: A national report*, March 2005, London: HO.

HO (2005b) *Consultation on the possession of extreme pornographic material*, London: HO.

HO (2006) *A coordinated prostitution strategy and a summary of responses to paying the price*, London: HO.

HO (2007a) *Review of the protection of children from sex offenders*, London: COI.

HO (2007b) *UK action plan on human trafficking*, London: HO.

HO (2008) *Violent crime action plan 2008–2011*, London: HO. Available HTTP: http://www.crimereduction.homeoffice.gov.uk/tvapshtvap002a2.pdf (accessed 10 February 2010).

HO (2009a) 'National domestic violence delivery plan 2009–10', in *National domestic violence delivery plan: annual progress report 2008–09*, London: HO.

HO (2009b) *Together we can end violence against women and girls: A strategy*, London: HO.

HO (2009c) *Crime in England and Wales 2007/8*, London: HO.

Hollins, S. (1999) 'Remorse for being: Through the lens of learning disability', in M. Cox (ed.), *Remorse and reparation*, London: Jessica Kingsley.

Hollins, S. and Grimer, M. (1988) *Going somewhere: Pastoral care for people with learning disabilities*, London: SPCK.

Hollins, S. and Sinason, V. (2000) 'Psychotherapy, learning disabilities and trauma: New perspectives', *British Journal of Psychiatry*, 176: 32–6.

Holt, S., Buckley, H. and Whelan, S. (2008) 'The impact of exposure to domestic violence on children and young people: A review of the literature', *Child Abuse and Neglect*, 32(8): 797–810.

Horner-Johnson, W. and Drum, C. (2006) 'Prevalence of maltreatment of people with intellectual disabilities: A review of recently published research', *Mental Retardation and Developmental Disabilities Research Reviews*, 12(1): 57–69.

Humphreys, C. and Thiara, R. (2002) *Routes to safety: Protection issues facing abused women and children and the role of outreach services*, Bristol: Women's Aid Federation of England.

Husain, M.I., Waheed, W. and Husain, N. (2006) 'Self-harm in British South Asian women: Psychosocial correlates and strategies for prevention', *Annuals of General Psychiatry*, 5: 1–7.

Isaac, A., Lockhart, L., and Williams, L. (2001) 'Violence against African American women in prisons and jails: Who's minding the shop?' *Journal of Human Behavior in the Social Environment*, 4(2/3): 129–53.

Island, D., and Letellier, P. (1991) *Men who beat the men who love them*, New York: Harrington Park Press.

Itzin, C. (ed.) (2000a) *Home truths about child sexual abuse: Influencing policy and practice – a reader*, London: Routledge.

Itzin, C. (2000b) 'Child protection and child sexual abuse prevention: influencing policy and practice', in C. Itzin (ed.), *Home truths about child sexual abuse: Influencing policy and practice – a reader*, London: Routledge.

Itzin, C. (2000c) 'Gendering domestic violence: The influence of feminism on policy and practice' in J. Hanmer and C. Itzin (eds), *Home truths about domestic violence: Feminist influences on policy and practice – a reader*, London: Routledge.

Itzin, C. (2002) 'Pornography and the construction of misogyny', *Journal of Sexual Aggression*, 8(3): 4–42.

Itzin, C. (2006) *Tackling the health and mental health effects of domestic and sexual violence and abuse*, London: Department of Health and Home Office.

Itzin, C., Taket, A. and Kelly, L. (2007) *The evidence of harm to adults relating to exposure to extreme pornographic material: A rapid evidence assessment*, London: Ministry of Justice Research Series 11/07. Available HTTP: http://www.justice.gov.uk/publications/research280907.htm (accessed 9 November 2009).

Jackson, E. (2010) *The end of my world*, London: Ebury Press.

Jacobson, A. (1989) 'Physical and sexual assault histories among psychiatric outpatients', *American Journal of Psychiatry*, 146: 755–8.

Jacobson, A. and Richardson, B. (1987) 'Assault experiences of 100 psychiatric inpatients: Evidence of the need for routine enquiry', *American Journal of Psychiatry*, 144: 908–13.

James-Hanman, D. (1998) *Social exclusion and domestic violence*, London: Greater London Domestic Violence Project.

Jaspard, M., Brown, E., Condon, S., Fougeyrollas-Schwebel, D., Houel, A., Lhomond, B., Maillochon, F., Saurel-Cubizolles, M.-J. and Schiltz, M.-A. (2003) *Les violences envers les femmes en France: un enquête nationale*, Paris: La Documentation française.

Jenny, C., Christian, C. W., Hibbard, R. A., Kellogg, N. D., Spivack, B. S., Stirling, J., Albers, L. M. H., Hermon, D. A. and Mason, P. W. (2008) 'Understanding the behavioural and emotional consequences of child abuse', *Pediatrics*, 122(3): 667–73.

Jespersen, A.F., Lalumiere, M.L. and Seto, M.C. (2009) 'Sexual abuse history among adult sex offenders and non-sex offenders: A meta-analysis', *Child Abuse and Neglect*, 33(3): 179–92.

Johnson, M.P. (2006) 'Conflict and control: Gender symmetry and asymmetry in domestic violence', *Violence Against Women*, 12: 1003–18.

Johnson, M.P. (2008) *A typology of domestic violence: intimate terrorism, violent resistance and situational couple violence*, Boston, MA: Northeastern University Press.

Kelly, L. (2000) 'Wars against women: Sexual violence, sexual politics and the militarised state', in S. Jacobs, R. Jacobson, and J. Marchbank (eds), *States of conflict: Gender, violence and resistance*, London: Zed Books.

Kelly, L., Regan, L., and Burton, S. (1991) *An exploratory study of the prevalence of sexual abuse in a sample of 16–21 year olds*, London: Child Abuse Studies Unit, University of North London.

Kemp, A., Dunstan, F., Harrison, S., Morris, S., Mann, M., Rolfe, K., Datta, S., Thomas, D.P., Sibert, J.R. and Maguire, S. (2008) 'Patterns of skeletal fractures in child abuse: Systematic review', *British Medical Journal*, 337: a1518.

Kendall-Tackett, K.A., Williams, L.M. and Finkelhor, D. (1993) 'Impact of sexual abuse on children: A review and synthesis of recent empirical studies', *Psychological Bulletin*, 113: 164–80.

Kendrick, A., and Taylor, J. (2000) 'Hidden on the ward: The abuse of children in hospitals', *Journal of Advanced Nursing*, 31(3), 565–73.

Kim, J. (2008) 'The protective effects of religiosity on maladjustment among mal-treated and nonmaltreated children', *Child Abuse and Neglect*, 32(7): 711–20.

Kimmel, M. (2002) 'Gender symmetry in domestic violence. A substantive and methodological research review', *Violence Against Women*, 8: 1332–63.

Kisiel, C.L. and Lyons, J.S. (2001) 'Dissociation as a mediator of psychopathology among sexually abused children and adolescents', *American Journal of Psychiatry*, 158: 1034–9.

Kitzmann, K.M., Gaylord, N.K., Noni, K., Holt, A.R. and Kenny, E.D. (2003) 'Child witnesses to domestic violence: A meta-analytic review', *Journal of Consulting and Clinical Psychology*, 71 (2): 339–52.

Kluft, R. (1990) 'Incest and subsequent revictimization: The case of therapist-patient sexual exploitation, with a description of the sitting duck syndrome', *Incest-related syndromes of adult psychopathology*, Washington, DC: American Psychiatric Association.

Knapp, J.F. (1998) 'The impact of children witnessing violence', *Pediatric Clinics of North America*, 45: 355–64.

Kolbo, J.R., Blakely, E.H. and Engleman, D. (1996) 'Children who witness domestic violence: A review of empirical literature', *Journal of Interpersonal Violence*, 11(2): 281–93.

Korf, D.J., Mot, E., Meulenbeek, H., and van den Brandt, T. (1997) *Economic costs of domestic violence against women, English summary of Economische kosten van thuisgeweld tegen vrouwen*, Utrecht: Stichting Vrouwenopvang Nederland.

Krahe, B., Bieneck, S. and Möller, I. (2005) 'Understanding gender and intimate partner violence from an international perspective', *Sex Roles: A Journal of Research*, 52(11–12): 807–27.

Krug, E.G., Dahlberg, L.L., Mercy, J.A., Zwi, A.B. and Lozano, R. (eds.) (2002) *World report on violence and health*, Geneva: World Health Organization.

Kumar, S. (2000) 'Client empowerment in psychiatry and the professional abuse of clients: Where do we stand?', *International Journal of Psychiatry in Medicine*, 30(1): 61–70.

Kvam, M.H. (2004) 'Sexual abuse of deaf children: A retrospective analysis of the prevalence and characteristics of childhood sexual abuse among deaf adults in Norway', *Child Abuse and Neglect*, 28(3): 241–51.

Lahm, K. (2009) 'Physical and property victimization behind bars', *International Journal of Offender Therapy and Comparative Criminology*, 53(3): 348–65.

Langevin, R., Curnoe, S. and Bain, J. (2000) 'A study of clerics who commit sexual offenses: Are they different from other sex offenders?' *Child Abuse and Neglect*, 24(4): 535–45.

Langstrom, N. (2001) *Young sex offenders: A research overview*, Stockholm, Sweden: The Board of Health and Welfare. Available HTTP: http://www.socialstyrelsen.se/Lists/Artikelkatalog/Attach-ments/11433/2001-123-17_200112317.pdf (accessed 9 November 2009).

Lansford, J.E., Dodge, K.A., Pettit, G.S., Bates, J.E., Crozier, J. and Kaplow, J. (2002) 'A 12-year prospective study of the long-term effects of early child physical maltreatment on psychological, behavioral, and academic problems in adolescence', *Archives of Pediatrics and Adolescent Medicine*, 156: 824–30.

Larkin, W. and Read, J. (2008) 'Childhood trauma and psychosis: Evidence, pathways and implications', *Journal of Postgraduate Medicine*, 54(4): 287–93.

Latthe, P., Mignini, L., Gray, R., Hills, K. and Khan, K. (2006) 'Factors predisposing women to chronic pelvic pain: Systematic review', *British Medical Journal*, 332(7544): 749–55.

Laws, D.R., and Marshall, W.L. (1990) 'A conditioning theory of the etiology and maintenance of deviant sexual preference and behaviour', in W. L. Marshall, D. R. Laws and H. E. Barbaree (eds.), *Handbook of sexual assault: Issues, theories, and treatment of the offender*, New York: Plenum Press.

Lay, M. and Papadopoulos, I. (2009) 'Sexual maltreatment of unaccompanied asylum-seeking minors from the Horn of Africa: A mixed methods study focusing on vulnerability and prevention', *Child Abuse and Neglect*, 33: 728–38.

Leeners, B., Richter-Appelt, H., Imthurn, B. and Rath, W. (2006) 'Influence of childhood sexual abuse on pregnancy, delivery and the early post-partum period in adult women', *Journal of Psychosomatic Research*, 61(2): 139–51.

Levitt, H.M. and Ware, K. (2006) ' "Anything with two heads is a monster": Religious leaders' perspectives on marital equality and domestic violence', *Violence Against Women*, 12(12): 1169–90.

Light, D. and Monk-Turner, E. (2009) 'Circumstances surrounding male sexual assault and rape: Findings from the national violence against women survey', *Journal of Interpersonal Violence*, 24(11): 1849–58.

Lindsay, W.R. (2002) 'Research and literature on sex offenders with intellectual and developmental disabilities', *Journal of Intellectual Disability Research*, 46(1): 74–85.

Lobel, K. (ed.) (1986) *Naming the violence: Speaking out about lesbian battering*, Seattle: Seal Press.

Lodewijks, H.P.B., de Ruiter, C. and Doreleijers, T.A.H. (2010) 'The impact of protective factors in desistance from violent reoffending: A study in three samples of adolescent offenders', *Journal of Interpersonal Violence*, 25(3): 568–87.

Losel, F. and Schmucker, M. (2005) 'The effectiveness of treatment for sexual offenders: A comprehensive meta-analysis', *Journal of Experimental Criminology*, 1: 117–46.

Lovell, E. (2002) *I think I may need some help with this problem: Responding to children and young people who display sexually harmful behaviours*, London: NSPCC.

Lucas, D.R., Wezner, K.C., Milner, J.S., McCanne, T.R., Harris, I.N., Monroe-Posey, C. and Nelson J.P. (2002) 'Victim, perpetrator, family, and incident characteristics of infant and child homicide in the United States Air Force', *Child Abuse and Neglect*, 26(2): 167–86.

Lundgren, E., Heimer, G., Westerstrand, J. and Kollikoski, A. (2002) *Captured Queen: Men's violence against women in 'equal' Sweden: A prevalence study*, Stockholm: Fritzes Offentliga Publikationer.

Luthra, R., Abramovitz, R., Greenberg, R., Schoor, A., Newcorn, J., Schmeidler, J., Levine, P., Nomura, Y. and Chemtob, C.M. (2009) 'Relationship between type of trauma exposure and posttraumatic stress disorder among urban children and adolescents', *Journal of Interpersonal Violence*, 24(11): 1919–27.

Lynch, M.A. (1975) 'Ill health and child abuse', *Lancet*, 2: 317–19.

McCarry, M., Hester, M. and Donovan, C. (2008) 'Researching same sex domestic violence: Constructing a survey methodology', *Sociological Research Online*, 13 (1). Online. Available HTTP: <http://www.socresonline.org.uk/13/1/8.html> (accessed 9 November 2009).

McClennen, J.C. (2005) 'Domestic violence between same-gender partners: Recent findings and future research', *Journal of Interpersonal Violence*, 20 (2): 149–54.

Macdonald, G.M., Higgins, J.P.T. and Ramchandani, P. (2006) 'Cognitive-behavioural interventions for children who have been sexually abused' *Cochrane Database of Systematic Reviews 2006*, Issue 4. Art. No.: CD001930. DOI: 10.1002/14651858.CD001930.pub2.

McDuff, E. (2008) 'Organizational context and the sexual harassment of clergy', *Sociology of Religion*, 69(3): 297–316.

Macfie, J., Cicchetti, D. and Toth, S.L. (2001) 'Dissociation in maltreated versus non-maltreated preschool-aged children', *Child Abuse and Neglect*, 25: 1253–67.

McGee, C. (2000a) *Childhood experiences of domestic violence*, London: Jessica Kingsley.

McGee, C. (2000b) 'Children's and mothers' experiences of support and protection following domestic violence', in J. Hanmer and C. Itzin (eds), *Home truths about domestic violence: Feminist influences on policy and practice – a reader*, London: Routledge.

McGloin, J.M. and Widom, C.S. (2001) 'Resilience among abused and neglected children grown up', *Development and Psychopathology*, 13: 1021–38.

MacKinnnon, C. (1987) *Feminism unmodified*, London: Harvard University Press.

MacMillan, H.L. with the Canadian Task Force on Preventive Health Care (2000) 'Preventive health care, 2000 update: Prevention of child maltreatment', *Canadian Medical Association Journal*, 163(11): 1451–8.

MacMillan, H.L., Wathen, C. N., Jamieson, E., Boyle, M.H., Shannon, H.S., Ford-Gilboe, M., Worster, A., Lent, B., Coben, J.H., Campbell, J.C. and McNutt, L. (2009) 'Screening for intimate partner violence in health care settings: A randomized trial', *Journal of the American Medical Association*, 302(5): 493–501.

McNeish, D. and Scott, S. (2008) *Mental health trusts collaboration project: Meeting the needs of survivors of abuse 3. Overview of evaluation findings September 2006 to July 2008*, Whitchurch: DMSS Research & Consultancy.

McQueen, D., Itzin, C., Kennedy, R., Sinason, V. and Maxted, F. (2008) *Psychoanalytic psychotherapy after child abuse, the treatment of adults and children who have experienced sexual abuse, violence and neglect in childhood*, London: Karnac.

McWilliams, M. and McKiernan, J. (1993) *Bringing it out into the open: Domestic violence in Northern Ireland*, London: HMSO.

Magowan, P. (2003) 'Domestic violence and disabled women', *Safe*, Bristol: Women's Aid, Spring 2003.

Mandell, D.S., Walrath,C.M., Manteuffel,B., Sgro,G. and Pinto-Martin,J.A. (2005) 'The prevalence and correlates of abuse among children with autism service in comprehensive community-based mental health settings', *Child Abuse and Neglect*, 29: 1359–72.

Marchant, R. (2008) 'Working with disabled children who live away from home some or all of the time', in M. Lefevre and B. Luckock (eds), *Direct work with children in care*, London: BAAF.

Marchant, R. (2009) 'Assessing children with complex needs', in J. Horwarth (ed.), *The child's world*, London: Jessica Kingsley.

Marchant, R. and Jones, M. (1999) 'Practice guidance for assessing disabled children and their families', in DH, *The framework for the assessment of children in need and their families*, London: DH.

Marchant, R. and Jones, M. (2008) '21 years of policy for disabled children', in *As long as it takes*, London: Action for Children.

Marchant, R., Lefevre, M., Luckock, B. and Jones, M. (2007) *The social care needs of children with complex health care needs*, London: Social Care Institute of Excellence.

Marcotte, D. (2008) 'The role of social factors in sexual misconduct of Roman Catholic clergy: A second look at John Jay data', *Sexual Addiction and Compulsivity*, 15: 23–8.

Marks, D. (2000) *Disability: Controversial debates and psychosocial perspectives*, London: Routledge.

Maxfield, M.G. and Widom, C.S. (1996) 'The cycle of violence: Revisited 6 years later', *Archives of Pediatrics and Adolescent Medicine*, 150: 390–5.

May-Chahal, C. and Cawson, P. (2005) 'Measuring child maltreatment in the United Kingdom: A study of the prevalence of child abuse and neglect', *Child Abuse and Neglect*, 29: 969–84.

Mays, J.M. (2006) 'Feminist disability theory: Domestic violence against women with a disability', *Disability and Society*, 21(2): 147–58.

Melhuish, E., Jay, B., Anning, A., Ball, M., Barnes, J., Romaniuk, H., Leyland, A. and the NESS Research Team (2007) 'Variation in community intervention programmes and consequences for children and families: The example of Sure Start Local Programme', *Journal of Child Psychology and Psychiatry*, 48(6): 543–51.

Melhuish, E., Belsky, J. Leyland, A. H., Barnes, J. and the NESS Research Team (2008) 'Effects of fully-established Sure Start Local Programmes on 3-year-old children and their families living in England: A quasi-experimental observational study', *Lancet* 372(9650): 1641–7.

Mencap (2007) *Bullying wrecks lives: The experiences of children and young people with a learning disability*, London: Mencap. Available HTTP: <http://www.mencap.org.uk/document.asp?id=164> (accessed 5 November 2009).

Messerschmidt, J. (2005) 'Men, Masculinities, and Crime', in M. Kimmel, R.W. Connell, and J. Hearn (eds), *Handbook on men and masculinities*, Thousand Oaks, CA: Sage.

Miller, S.L. (2001) 'The paradox of women arrested for domestic violence', *Violence Against Women*, 7: 1339–76.

Miller, S.L. and Meloy, M.L. (2006) 'Women's use of force: Voices of women arrested for domestic violence', *Violence Against Women*, 12: 89–115.

Mirlees-Black, C. (1999) *Domestic violence: Findings from a new British crime survey self completion questionnaire, Home Office Research Study 191*, London: Home Office Publications.

Mooney, A., Owen, C. and Statham, J. (2008) *Disabled children: Numbers, characteristics and local service provision*, London: Thomas Coram Research Unit, Institute of Education, University of London.

Mooney, J. (1994) *The hidden figure: Domestic violence in North London*, London: Islington Police and Crime Prevention Unit.

Mooney, J. (2000) 'Revealing the hidden figure of domestic violence', in J. Hanmer, and C. Itzin (eds), *Home truths about domestic violence: Feminists influences on policy and practice*, London: Routledge.

Moran, L. and Skeggs, B. (2004) *Sexuality and the politics of violence and safety*, London: Routledge.

Morgan, S.R. (1987) *Abuse and neglect of handicapped children*, Boston, MA: College-Hill Publication, Little Brown and Company.

Moster, A. and Jeglic, E. (2009) 'Prison warden attitudes toward prison rape and sexual assault: Findings since the Prison Rape Elimination Act (PREA)', *The Prison Journal*, 89(1): 65–78.

Mullender, A. (1996) *Rethinking domestic violence: the social work and probation response*, London: Routledge.

Mullender, A., Hague, G., Imam, U., Kelly, L., Malos, L. and Regan, L. (2002) *Children's perspectives on domestic violence*, London: Routledge.

Müller, U. and Schröttle, M. (2004) *Lebenssituation, Sicherheit und Gesundheit von Frauen in Deutschland: eine repräsentative untersuchung zu gewalt gegen frauen in Deutschland*, Berlin: Zusammenfassung zentraler Studiengergebnisse, Bundesministerium für Familie, Frauen und Jugend.

Murdoch, M., and Nichol, K. (1995) 'Women veterans' experiences with domestic violence and with sexual harassment while in the military', *Archives of Family Medicine*, 4(5): 411–18.

Murphy, C.C., Schei, B., Myhr, T.L. and Du Mont, J. (2001) 'Abuse: a risk factor for low birth weight? A systematic review and meta-analysis', *Canadian Medical Association Journal*, 164: 1567–72.

Murray, M. and Osborne, C. (2009) *Safeguarding disabled children: Practice guidance*, London: DCSF.

National Autistic Society (2006) *B is for Bullied: Experiences of children with autism and their families*, London: National Autistic Society.

Nayak, M.B., Byrne, C.A., Martin, M.K. and Abraham, A.G. (2003) 'Attitudes toward violence against women: A cross-nation study', *Sex Roles*, 49(7–8): 333–42.

NCCWCH (National Collaborating Centre for Women's and Children's Health) (2009) *When to suspect child maltreatment, commissioned by the National Institute for Health and Clinical Excellence*, London: RCOG Press.

NCIPC (2003) *Costs of intimate partner violence against women in the United States*, Atlanta, GA: National Centre for Injury Prevention and Control, Centers for Disease Prevention and Control.

Neigh, G.N., Gillespie, C.F. and Nemeroff, C.B. (2009) 'The neurobiological toll of child abuse and neglect', *Trauma, Violence and Abuse*, 10(4): 389–410.

Nelson, H.D., Nygren, P., McInerney, Y. and Klein, J. (2004) 'Screening women and elderly adults for family and intimate partner violence: A review of the evidence for the U.S. preventative services task force', *Annals of Internal Medicine*, 140(5): 387–404.

NICE (2004) *Guidelines on self harm*, London: National Institute for Health and Clinical Excellence.

NICE (2008) *Promoting children's social and emotional wellbeing in primary education: NICE public health guidance 12*, London: National Institute for Health and Clinical Excellence.

NICE (2009) *Promoting children's social and emotional wellbeing in secondary education: NICE public health guidance 20*, London: National Institute for Health and Clinical Excellence.

Noll, J.G., Trickett, P.K., Harris, W.W. and Putnam, F.W. (2009) 'The cumulative burden borne by offspring whose mothers were sexually abused as children: Descriptive results from a multigenerational study', *Journal of Interpersonal Violence*, 24(3): 424–49.

Nosek, M.A. and Howland, C.A. (1998) *Abuse and women with disabilities*, Harrisburg, PA: National Online Resource Center on Violence Against Women, Pennsylvania Coalition Against Domestic Violence.

Nosek, M.A., Howland, C.A. and Young, M.E. (1997) 'Abuse of women with disabilities: Policy implications', *Journal of Disability Policy Studies*, 8: 157–76.

Nosek, M.A., Howland, C.A. and Hughes, R.B. (2001) 'The investigation of abuse and women with disabilities: Going beyond assumptions', *Violence Against Women*, 7(4): 477–99.

Nosek, M.A., Hughes, R.B., Taylor, H. and Taylor, P. (2006) 'Disability, psychosocial and demographic characteristics of abused women with physical disabilities', *Violence Against Women*, 12(9): 838–50.

Nurse, J. (2006) *Preventing Violence and Abuse: Creating safe and respectful lives*, South East Regional Public Health Group Information Series 1, London: DH and HO.

O'Donnell, I. and Edgar, K. (1998) 'Routine victimisation in prisons', *Howard Journal of Criminal Justice*, 37(3): 266–79.

O'Driscoll, D. (2009) 'Psychotherapy and intellectual disability: A historical view', in T. Cottis (ed.), *Intellectual disability, trauma and psychotherapy*, London: Routledge.

O'Neill, W.L. (1998) 'Sex scandals in the gender-integrated military', *Gender Issues*, 16(1): 64–86.

O'Reilly, R. (2007) 'Domestic violence against women in their childbearing years: A review of the literature', *Contemporary Nurse*, 25(1-2): 13–21.

Office of the Children's Commissioner (2006) *Bullying today: A report by the Office of the Children's Commissioner*, London: OCC.

Olff, M., Langeland, W., Draijer, N., and Gersons, B.P.R. (2007) 'Gender differences in posttraumatic stress disorder', *Psychological Bulletin*, 133(2): 183–204.

Oliver, J. (1988) 'Successive generations of child maltreatment', *British Journal of Psychiatry*, 153: 543–53.

Oliver, C., Murphy, G., and Corbett, J. (1987) 'Self-injurious behaviour in people with mental handicaps: A total population study', *Journal of Mental Deficiency Research*, 31: 147–62.

Olver, M.E., Wong, S.C.P and Nicholaichuk, T.P. (2009) 'Outcome evaluation of a high-intensity inpatient sex offender treatment program', *Journal of Interpersonal Violence*, 24(3): 522–36.

Pan, A., Rivera, L., Lingle, D., Williams, K., Griffin-Tabor, V. and Reznik, V. (2003) 'Lessons learned from the Ahimsa Project: Domestic violence in Latino, Somali and Vietnamese communities of San Diego'. Paper presented at American Public Health Association conference, San Francisco, November, 2003.

Paolucci, E.O., Genuis, M. L. and Violato, C. (2001) 'A meta-analysis of the published research on the effects of child sexual abuse', *Journal of Psychology*, 135(1): 17–36.

Payne, S. (2004) 'Sex, gender and irritable bowel syndrome: Making the connections', *Gender Medicine*, 1(1): 18–28.

Payne, S. (2006) *The health of men and women*, London: Polity Press.

Peleikis, D.E. and Dahl, A.A. (2005) 'A systematic review of empirical studies of psychotherapy with women who were sexually abused as children', *Psychotherapy Research*, 15(3): 304–15.

Pereda, N., Guilera, G., Forns, M. and Gomez-Benito, J. (2009) 'The international epidemiology of child sexual abuse: A continuation of Finkelhor (1994)', *Child Abuse and Neglect*, 33: 331–42.

POPAN (2004) *Ten years is too long: Proposals for interim public protection measures in the talking therapies*. Available at HTTP: <http://www.popan.org.uk/policy/documents/TenYearsIsTooLong.pdf> (accessed 9 November 2009).

Povey, D. (ed.), Coleman, K., Kaiza, P., Hoare, J. and Jansson, K. (2008) *Homicides, firearm offences and intimate violence 2006/07 (Supplementary Volume 2 to Crime in England and Wales 2006/07)*, London: Home Office Statistical Bulletin 3/08. Available HTTP: <http://www.homeoffice.gov.uk/rds/pdfs08/hosb0308.pdf> (accessed 9 November 2009).

Price, J.L., Hilsenroth, M.J., Petretic-Jackson, P.A. and Bonge, D. (2001) 'A review of individual psychotherapy outcomes for adult survivors of childhood sexual abuse', *Clinical Psychology Review*, 21(7): 1095–121.

Print, B. and Morrison, T. (2000) 'Treating adolescents who sexually abuse others', in C. Itzin (ed.), *Home truths about child sexual abuse: Influencing policy and practice – a reader*, London: Routledge.

Pritchard, J. (2000) *The needs of older women: Services for victims of elder abuse and other abuse*, Bristol: The Policy Press.

Putnam, F.W. (2003) 'Ten-year research update review: Child sexual abuse', *Journal of the American Academy of Child and Adolescent Psychiatry*, 42(3): 269–78.

Radford, J., Harne, L. and Trotter, J. (2005) *Good intentions – Disabling realities: Disabled women experiencing domestic violence*, Middlesbrough: Middlesbrough Domestic Violence Forum.

Radford, J., Harne, L. and Trotter, J. (2006) 'Disabled women and domestic violence as violent crime in practice', *Journal of the British Association of Social Workers*, 18(4): 233–46.

Raiha, N., and Soma, D. (1997) 'Victims of child abuse and neglect in the US Army', *Child Abuse and Neglect*, 21(8): 759–68.

Raleigh, V.S. (1996) 'Suicide patterns and trends in people of Indian sub-continent and Caribbean origin in England and Wales', *Ethnicity and Health*, 1(1): 55–63.

Ramchandani, P. and Jones, D.P.H. (2003) 'Treating psychological symptoms in sexually abused children: From research findings to service provision', *British Journal of Psychiatry*, 183: 484–90.

Ramsay, J., Richardson, J., Carter, Y.H., Davidson, L.L. and Feder, G. (2002) 'Should health professionals screen women for domestic violence? Systematic review', *British Medical Journal*, 325: 314–27.

Ramsay, J., Rivas, C. and Feder, G. (2005) *Interventions to reduce violence and promote the physical and psychological well-being of women who experience partner violence: a systematic review of controlled evaluations. Final Report*, London: Barts and The London Queen Mary's School of Medicine and Dentistry.

RCP (2004) *Council Report 116*, London: Royal College of Psychiatry.

Read, J., Clements, L. and Ruebain, D. (2006) *Disabled children and the law* (2nd edn), London: JKP.

Read, J., Spencer, N. and Blackburn, C. (2008) *Can we count them? Disabled children and their households*, Coventry: University of Warwick.

Reid, R.J., Bonomi, A.E., Rivara, F.P., Anderson, M.L., Fishman, P.A., Carrell, D.S. and Thompson, R.S. (2008) 'Intimate partner violence among men: Prevalence, chronicity and health effects', *American Journal of Preventative Medicine*, 34(6): 478–85.

Reitzel, L.R. and Carbonell, J.L. (2006) 'The effectiveness of sexual offender treat-ment for juveniles as measured by recidivism: A meta-analysis' *Sexual Abuse: A Journal of Research and Treatment*, 18(4): 401–21.

Rentz, E., Martin, S., Gibbs, D., Clinton-Sherrod, M., Hardison, J. and Marshall, S. (2006) 'Family violence in the military: A review of the literature', *Trauma, Violence and Abuse*, 7(2): 93–108.

Renzetti, C. (1992) *Violent betrayal: Partner abuse in lesbian relationships*, Newbury Park, CA: Sage.

Respect (2004) *Statement of principles and minimum standards of practice for domestic violence perpetrator programmes and associated women's services*, London: Respect.

Ricks, D. (1990) 'Mental handicap', in H. Wolff, A. Bateman, and D. Sturgeon (eds), *UCH textbook of psychiatry*, London: Duckworth.

Rieser, R. and Mason, M. (1992) 'Disability equality in the classroom: A human rights issue', in G. Thomas and M. Vaughan (eds), (2004) *Inclusive education: Readings and reflections*, Maidenhead: Open University Press.

Ristock, J. (2002) *No more secrets: Violence in lesbian relationships*, London: Routledge.

Roberto, K., and Teaster, P. (2005) 'Sexual abuse of vulnerable young and old women', *Violence Against Women*, 11(4): 473–502.

Rodgers, S. (1995) 'Health care providers and sexual assault: Feminist law reform?', *Canadian Journal of Women & the Law*, 8(1): 159–89.

Romito, P., Turan, J.M. and De Marchi, M. (2005) 'The impact of current and past interpersonal violence on women's mental health', *Social Science and Medicine*, 60: 1717–27.

Roodman, A.A. and Clum, G.A. (2001) 'Revictimization rates and method variance: A meta-analysis', *Clinical Psychology Review*, 21(2): 183–204.

Rosenberg, M.S. and Rossman, B.B. (1990) 'The child witness to marital violence', in A.T. Ammerman and M. Herson (eds), *Treatment of family violence*, New York: John Wiley and Sons.

Roth, S. and Cohen, L.J. (1986) 'Approach, avoidance and coping with stress', *American Psychologist*, 41(7): 813–19.

Russell, D.E. and Bolen, R.M. (2000) *The epidemic of rape and child sexual abuse in the United States*, Thousand Oaks, CA: Sage.

Rutter, M., Tizard, J. and Whitmore, K. (1970) *Education, health and behaviour*, London: Longman.

Sands, K.M. (2003) 'Speaking out: Clergy sexual abuse: where are the women?' *Journal of Feminist Studies in Religion*, 19(2): 79–83.

Sarkar, N.N. and Sarkar, R. (2005) 'Sexual assault on woman: Its impact on her life and living in society', *Sexual and Relationship Therapy*, 20(4): 407–19.

Saunders, D.G. (2002) 'Are physical assaults by wives and girlfriends a major social problem? A review of the literature', *Violence Against Women*, 8 (12): 1424–48.

Saunders, B.E., Berliner, L. and Hanson, R.F. (eds.), (2004). *Child physical and sexual abuse: Guidelines for treatment, revised report: April 26, 2004*, Charleston, SC: National Crime Victims Research and Treatment Center.

Saxton, M., Curry, M.A., Powers, L., Maley, S., Eckels, K. and Gross, J. (2001) 'Bring my scooter so I can leave you: A study of disabled women handling abuse by personal assistance providers', *Violence Against Women*, 7: 393–417.

SBS (forthcoming) *Safe and sane: A model of intervention on domestic violence and mental health, suicide and self-harm amongst black and minority ethnic women*, London: SBS.

Schultz, D., Tharp-Taylor, S. Haviland, A. and Jaycox, L. (2009) 'The relationship between protective factors and outcomes for children investigated for maltreatment', *Child Abuse and Neglect*, 33(10): 684–98.

Shadigian, E.M. and Bauer, S.T. (2005) 'Pregnancy-associated death: A qualitative systematic review of homicide and suicide', *Obstetrical and Gynecological Survey*, 60(3): 183–90.

Shankleman, J., Brooks, R. and Webb, E. (2001) *Children resident in domestic violence refuges in Cardiff: A health needs and healthcare needs assessment*, Cardiff: University of Cardiff, Department of Child Health.

Sharpen, J. (2009) *Improving safety, reducing harm, children, young people and domestic violence: A practical toolkit for front-line practitioners*, London: DH.

Shorey, R.C., Cornelius, T.L. and Bell, K.M. (2008) 'A critical review of theoretical frameworks for dating violence: Comparing the dating and marital fields', *Aggression and Violent Behaviour*, 13: 185–94.

Silva, C., McFarlane, J., Soeken, K., Parker, B. and Reel, S. (1997) 'Symptoms of post-traumatic stress disorder in abused women in a primary care setting', *Journal of Women's Health*, 6: 543–52.

Silverman, J.G., Raj, A. and Clements, K. (2004) 'Dating violence and associated sexual risk and pregnancy among adolescent girls in the United States', *Pediatrics*, 114(2): 220–5.

Simon, T.R., Anderson, M., Thompson, M.P., Crosby, A.E., Shelley, G. and Sacks, J.J. (2001) 'Attitudinal acceptance of intimate partner violence among US adults', *Violence and Victims*, 16(2): 115–26.

Simons, D.A., Wurtele, S.K. and Durham, R.L. (2008) 'Developmental experiences of child abusers and rapists', *Child Abuse and Neglect*, 32: 549–60.

Sinason, V. (1991) 'Abuse and disability', paper, presented at the ACPP Study Day, London, 9 October 1991. Published as: Sinason, V. (1999) 'Abuse and disability', in C. Schwabenland (ed.), *Relationships in the lives of people with learning difficulties*, London: Elfrida Press.

Sinason, V. (1992a) *Mental handicap and the human condition: New approaches from the Tavistock*, London: Free Association Books.

Sinason, V. (1992b) 'Psychotherapy with profoundly handicapped children', in S. Ramsden (ed.), *Psychotherapy – pure and applied: Papers and workshops*, London: Association for Child Psychology and Psychiatry.

Sinason, V. (2004) 'Learning disability as a trauma and the impact of trauma on people with a learning disability', Unpublished PhD, London: St George's Hospital Medical School Mental Health Unit.

Skinner, K., Kressin, N., Frayne, S., Tripp, T., Hankin, C., Miller, D. and Sullivan, L.M. (2000) 'The prevalence of military sexual assault among female veterans' administration outpatients', *Journal of Interpersonal Violence*, 15(3): 291–310.

Slashinski, M.J., Coker, A.L. and Divs, K.E. (2003) 'Physical aggression, forced sex, and stalking victimization by a dating partner: An analysis of the National Violence Against Women Survey', *Violence and Victims*, 18(6): 595–617.

Smith, K. (ed.), Flatley, J. (ed.), Coleman, K., Osborne, S., Kaiza, P. and Roe, S. (2010) *Homicides, Firearms Offences and Intimate Violence 2008/09*. Home Office Statistical Bulletin 01/10, London: Home Office.

Smolak, L. and Murnen, S. K. (2002) 'A meta-analytic examination of the relation-ship between child sexual abuse and eating disorders', *International Journal of Eating Disorders*, 31(2): 136–50.

Sobsey, D. (2000) 'Faces of violence against women with disabilities', *Impact*, 13(3), Minnesota: Institute on Community Integration (UCEDD) and the Research Training Center on Community Living. Available: <http://ici.umn.edu/products/impact/133/default.html> (accessed 5 November 2009).

Social Exclusion Unit (2004) *Mental health and social exclusion*, London: Office of the Deputy Prime Minister.

Sox, R. (2004) 'Integrative review of recent child witness to violence research', *Clinical Excellence for Nurse Practitioners*, 8(2): 68–78.

Spitz, R. (1953) 'Aggression: Its role in the establishment of object relations', in R. Emde (ed.), *Dialogues from infancy*, New York: International Universities Press, 1983.

Stanko, B. (2003) 'Intentional violence in the UK: What the available data show', paper presented at National Launch of the WHO report, London: September 2003.

Stark, E. (2007) *Coercive control*, New York: Oxford University Press.

Stark, E. and Flitcraft, A. (1988) 'Women and children at risk: A feminist perspec-tive on child abuse', *International Journal of Health Services*, 18(1): 97–118.

Sternfeld, L. (1977) 'Report of the medical director to the members of the corpora-tion', paper presented at UCPA Annual Conference, Washington, DC, April.

Stith, S.M., Rosen, K.H., Middleton, K.A., Busch, A.L., Lundeberg, K. and Carlton, R.P. (2000) 'The intergenerational transmission of spouse abuse: A meta-analysis', *Journal of Marriage and the Family*, 62(3): 640–54.

Straus, M.A. (1999) 'The controversy over domestic violence by women: A meth-odological, theoretical, and sociology of science analysis', in X.B. Arriaga and S. Oskamp (eds), *Violence in intimate relationships*, Thousand Oaks, CA: Sage Publications.

Straus, M., Gelles, R. and Steinmetz, S. (1980) *Behind closed doors: Violence in the American family*, Newbury Park, CA: Sage.

Struckman-Johnson, C. and Struckman-Johnson, D. (2006) 'A comparison of sexual coercion experiences reported by men and women in prison', *Journal of Interper-sonal Violence*, 21(12): 1591–615.

Sullivan, P.M. (2003) 'Violence against children with disabilities: Prevention, public policy, and research implications', paper presented at National Conference on Preventing and Intervening in Violence Against Children and Adults with Disabili-ties, SUNY Upstate Medical University, NY, May 2002.

Sullivan, P. and Knutson, J. (1998) 'The association between child maltreatment and disabilities in a hospital-based epidemiological study', *Child Abuse and Neglect*, 22(4): 271–88.

Sullivan, P. and Knutson, J. (2000) 'Maltreatment and disabilities: A population-based epidemiological study', *Child Abuse and Neglect*, 24(10): 1257–73.

Sullivan, P., Vernon, M. and Scanlan, J. (1987) 'Sexual abuse of deaf youth', *American Annals of the Deaf*, 1: 256–62.

Swann, S. (2000) 'Helping girls involved in "prostitution" A Barnardos' experi-ment', in C. Itzin (ed.), *Home truths about child sexual abuse: Influencing policy and practice – a reader*, London: Routledge.

Taft, A., Hegarty, K. and Flood, M. (2001) 'Are men and women equally violent to intimate partners?' *Australian and New Zealand Journal of Public Health*, 25: 498–500.

Taket, A. and Barter-Godfrey, S. (2006) *Delphi expert consultation – Final Report. Report to Department of Health, Victims of Violence and Abuse Prevention Programme*, Melbourne: Deakin University.

Taket, A., Beringer, A., Irvine, A. and Garfield, S. (2004) *Tackling domestic violence: Exploring the health service contribution: evaluation of the Crime Reduction Programme Violence Against Women Initiative health projects*. Home Office Online Report 52/04. Available HTTP: <http://www.homeoffice.gov.uk/rds/pdfs04/rdsolr5204.pdf> (accessed 5 November 2009).

Taket, A., Crisp, B.R., Nevill, A., Lamaro, G., Graham, M. and Barter-Godfrey, S. (2009) *Theorising social exclusion*, London: Routledge.

Taylor, C.A. and Sorenson, S.B. (2003) 'Factors associated with normative beliefs about fault and taking responsibility for intimate partner violence', paper presented at American Public Health Association conference, San Francisco, November 2003.

Taylor, M. and Quayle, E. (2003) *Child pornography: An internet crime*, New York: Brunner-Routledge.

Thomas, S.P. and Hall J.M. (2008) 'Life trajectories of female child abuse survivors thriving in adulthood', *Qualitative Health Research*, 18(2): 149–66.

Titunik, R. (2009) 'Are we all torturers now? A reconsideration of women's violence at Abu Ghraib', *Cambridge Review of International Affairs*, 22(2): 257–77.

Tjaden, P. and Thoennes, N. (2000) *Full report of the prevalence, incidence and consequences of violence against women: Findings from the National Violence Against Women Survey*, Washington, DC: US Department of Justice.

Tjaden, P., Thoennes, N. and Allison, C.J. (1999) 'Comparing violence over the life span in samples of same sex and opposite cohabitants', *Violence and Victims*, 14(4): 413–25.

Todahl, J.L., Linville, D., Bustin, A., Wheeler, J. and Gau, J. (2009) 'Sexual assault support services and community systems: Understanding critical issues and needs in the LGBTQ community', *Violence Against Women*, 15(8): 952–76.

Topping, K. J. and Barron, I. G. (2009) 'School-based child sexual abuse prevention programs: A review of effectiveness', *Review of Educational Research*, 79(1): 431–63.

Tymchuk, A. and Andron, L. (1990) 'Mothers with mental retardation who do or do not abuse or neglect their children', *Child Abuse and Neglect*, 14 (3): 313–23.

UKP (2002) United Kingdom Parliament Adoption and Children Act chapter 38. Online. Available HTTP: <http://www.opsi.gov.uk/acts/acts2002/ukpga_20020038_en_1> (accessed 10 February 2010).

UKP (2003) United Kingdom Parliament Sexual Offences Act chapter 42. Online. Available HTTP: <http://www.opsi.gov.uk/acts/acts2003/ukpga_20030042_en_1> (accessed 10 February 2010).

UKP (2004) United Kingdom Parliament Domestic Violence, Crime and Victims Act chapter 28. Online. Available HTTP: <http://www.opsi.gov.uk/acts/acts2004/ukpga_20040028_en_1> (accessed 10 February 2010).

UKP (2006) United Kingdom Parliament Equality Act chapter 3. Online. Available HTTP: <http://www.opsi.gov.uk/acts/acts2003/ukpga_20030042_en_1> (accessed 10 February 2010).

UKP (2008) United Kingdom Parliament Criminal Justice and Immigration Act chapter 4. Online. Available HTTP: <http://www.opsi.gov.uk/acts/acts2008/ukpga_20080004_en_1> (accessed 10 February 2010).

UN (1995) Beijing Platform for Action. Online. Available HTTP: <http://www.un.org/womenwatch/daw/beijing/platform/> (accessed 10 February 2010).

UN (1996) Declaration on the Elimination of Violence Against Women. Online. Available HTTP: <http://www.un.org/rights/dpi1772e.htm> (accessed 10 February 2010).

UN (2005) Report of the Secretary-General's Special Advisor, Prince Zeid Ra'ad Zeid al-Hussein on 'A comprehensive strategy to eliminate future sexual exploitation and abuse in United Nations peacekeeping operations' (24 March 2005). Department of Peace Keeping Operations, United Nations. Available HTTP: <http://www.un.org/Depts/dpko/dpko/reports> (accessed 9 November 2009).

Ungar, M., Tutty, L.M., McConnell, S., Barter, K. and Fairholm, J. (2009) 'What Canadian youth tell us about disclosing abuse', *Child Abuse and Neglect*, 33: 699–708.

USCCB (2004) *The John Jay Report*, United States Conference of Catholic Bishops. Available HTTP: <http://www.usccb.org/nrb/johnjaystudy/> (accessed 9 November 2009).

Valente, S.M. (2005) 'Sexual abuse of boys', *Journal of Child and Adolescent Psychiatric Nursing*, 18(1): 10–16.

Valenti-Hein, D. and Schwartz, L. (1995) *The sexual abuse interview for those with developmental disabilities*, Santa Barbara: James Stanfield Company.

van Ineveld C.H., Cook D.J., Kane S.L. and King D. (1996) 'Discrimination and abuse in internal medicine residency', *Journal General Internal Medicine*, 11(7): 401–5.

Vandiver, D. and Teske, R. (2006) 'Juvenile female and male sex offenders', *International Journal of Offender Therapy and Comparative Criminology*, 50(2): 148–65.

Vanya, M. (2001) 'What Slovak women perceive to be domestic violence', *Sociologia*, 33(3): 275–96.

Veltman, M. W. M. and Browne, K. D. (2001) 'Three decades of child maltreatment research: Implications for the school years', *Trauma, Violence, and Abuse: A Review Journal*, 2(3): 215–39.

Verdugo, M.A., Bermejo, B.G. and Fuertes, J. (1995) 'The maltreatment of intellectually handicapped-children and adolescents', *Child Abuse and Neglect*, 19(2): 205–15.

Vizard, E., Hickey, N., French, L. and McCrory, E. (2007) 'Children and adolescents who present with sexually abusive behaviour: A UK descriptive study', *Journal of Forensic Psychiatry and Psychology*, 18(1): 59–73.

Walby, S. (2004) *The cost of domestic violence*, London: National Statistics, Department of Trade and Industry.

Walby, S. and Allen, J. (2004) *Domestic violence, sexual assault and stalking: Findings from the British Crime Survey*, Home Office Research Study 276, London: Home Office.

Walker, D.F., McGovern, S.K., Poey, E.L. and Otis, K.E. (2005) 'Treatment effectiveness for male adolescent sexual offenders: A meta-analysis and review', *Journal of Child Sexual Abuse*, 13(3): 281–93.

Ware, K., Levitt, H. and Bayer, G. (2003) 'May God help you: Faith leaders' perspectives of intimate partner violence within their communities', *Journal of Religion and Abuse*, 5(2): 55–81.

Wathen, C.N. and MacMillan, H.L. (2003) 'Interventions for violence against women: Scientific review', *Journal of the American Medical Association*, 289(5): 589–600.

Wells, R.D., McCann, J., Adams, J., Voris, J. and Ensign, J. (1995) 'Emotional, behavioral, and physical symptoms reported by parents of sexually abused, non-abused, and allegedly abused prepubescent females', *Child Abuse and Neglect*, 19:155–63.

Westmarland, N., Hester, M. and Reid, P. (2004) *Routine enquiry about domestic violence in GP practices: A pilot study,* Bristol: University of Bristol.

Whitaker, D. J., Le, B., Hanson, R. K., Baker, C. K., McMahon, P. M., Ryan, G., Klein, A. and Rice, D. D. (2008). 'Risk factors for the perpetration of child sexual abuse: A review and meta-analysis', *Child Abuse and Neglect,* 32(5): 529–48.

Whitaker, D. J., Morrison, S., Lindquist, C., Hawkins, S.R., O'Neil, J.A., Nesius, A.M., Mathew, A. and Reese, L.R. (2006) 'A critical review of interventions for the primary prevention of perpetration violence', *Aggression and Violent Behavior,* 11: 151–66.

Whittle, N., Bailey, S. and Kurz, Z. (2006) *The needs and effective treatment of young people who sexually abuse: current evidence,* London: Department of Health and Home Office.

WHO (1997) *Violence against women: A health priority issue, FRH/WHD/97.8,* Geneva: WHO.

Wilcox, D.T. (2004) 'Treatment of intellectually disabled individuals who have committed sexual offences: A review of the literature', *Journal of Sexual Agression,* 10(1): 85–100.

Williams, J. and Nash, J. (2001) 'Meeting the advocacy needs of people who have been abused by health and social care practitioners', *Journal of Community and Applied Social Psychology,* 11: 361–70.

Willis, B.M. and Levy, B.S. (2002) 'Child prostitution: Global health burden, research needs, and interventions', *Lancet,* 359: 1417–22.

Wither, J.K. (2004) 'Battling bullying in the British Army 1987–2004', *The Journal of Power Institutions in Post-Soviet Societies,* 1: 1–12.

Wolfe, D. A., Crooks, C. V., Lee, V., McIntyre-Smith, A. and Jaffe, P. (2003) 'The effects of children's exposure to domestic violence: A meta-analysis and critique', *Clinical Child and Family Psychology Review,* 6(3): 171–87.

Wolff, N., Shi, J. and Blitz, C. (2008) 'Racial and ethnic disparities in types and sources of victimization inside prison', *The Prison Journal,* 88(4): 451–72.

Wonderlich, S.A., Crosby, R.D., Mitchell, J.E., Roberts, J. A., Haseltine, B., DeMuth, G. and Thompson, K. M. (2000) 'Relationship of childhood sexual abuse and eating disturbance in children', *Journal of the American Academy of Child and Adolescent Psychiatry,* 39: 1277–83.

WWDA (2004) Submission to the South Australian Government's discussion paper: "Valuing South Australia's women: Towards a Safety Strategy for South Australia", Australia: WWDA. Online. Available HTTP: <http://www.wwda. org.au/saviolsub.htm> (accessed 5 November 2009).

Wyre, R. (2000) 'Paedophile characteristics and patterns of behaviour: developing and using a typology', in C. Itzin (ed.), *Home truths about child sexual abuse: Influencing policy and practice,* London: Routledge.

Yassi, A. (1994) 'Assault and abuse of health care workers in a large teaching hospital', *Canadian Medical Association Journal,* 151(9): 1273–9.

Zielinski, D.S. (2009) 'Child maltreatment and adult socioeconomic well-being', *Child Abuse and Neglect,* 33(10): 666–8.

Zimmerman, C., Hossain, M., Yun, K., Roche, B., Morison, L. and Watts, C. (2006) *Stolen smiles: A summary report on the physical and psychological health consequences of women and adolescents trafficked in Europe,* London: London School of Hygiene and Tropical Medicine.

Index